The Homemade Medicine Book
By Charles Silverman N.D.

I0500412

THE
Homemade
MEDICINE   BOOK
~ 3rd Edition ~

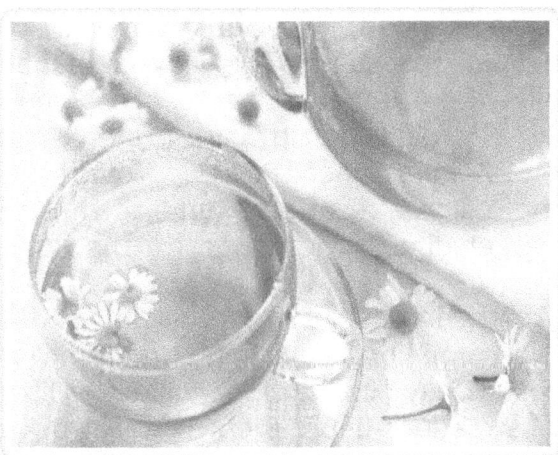

For the first time a Naturopathic Doctor opens his vault to unveil the complete list of home remedies used by professionals Holistic Practitioners...

Charles Silverman N.D.

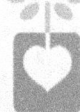

Introduction

We are all trying to go back to basics when it comes to our health, meaning we are going back to natural remedies like the ones used in homeopathy, herbal therapy, healing foods and home remedies.

All of them are part of what's called "alternative medicine." I'm sure you have heard of the tremendous success these techniques have accomplished in the past and all of them have been used for

more than 200 years.

When it comes to herbal treatment Americans are decades behind. Europe, China and India have used herbs for thousands of years. These countries have incorporated herbs into their conventional treatments and their pharmacies carry a wide array of herbal medicines. Herbs like Ginkgo Biloba have had more than 300 tests done in Germany and France. In the United States today federal law prohibits manufacturers of herbal products from marketing their remedies as medicines. Instead herbal remedies are sold as food products and their labels cannot mention or claim any disease fighting property unless they have received drug approval from FDA.

Manufacturers in Europe have very little problem getting their remedies certified for medical use. The industry is very well regulated and the process is cheaper and easier. This way of managing the health system has given the European citizens access to wide variety of medicines and to an affordable health care system. Meanwhile in the United States the FDA takes decades to approve synthetic drugs that still produce horrible side effects and some of these drugs have to be taken off the market due to the danger to the public.

But millions of Americans are catching on and getting tired of the massive advertising campaigns paid for by multimillion dollars laboratories, urging you to buy "something" for every little illness you may have, such as constipation, depression, headaches, toothaches, earaches, fever, insomnia or even a cold. And people are also learning that the drugs these labs are selling are full of side effects, and only mask symptoms, blocking the body's attempt to heal itself.

Nature has given us the most wonderful machine ever invented, our immune system. If we give it a chance it will heal by itself but often we abuse our body so much that even this perfect machine needs help. By giving our body the right nutrients and medicines we can bring our healing force back in balance with no expensive drugs that only treat the symptoms and not the disease.

TIP: An estimated 100,000 people are hospitalized and 16,000 die of side effects caused by arthritis drugs each year.

In this book you will find everything you need to better your health with herbs, nutrients, vitamins, exercise and healing using completely natural remedies.

We will tell you how to treat the most common ailments that affect us all. It is important to know that you don't have to run to the pharmacy every time something hurts or someone gets sick. Most of the illness that we encounter on a daily basis can be treated without expensive synthetic drugs.

We all have seen the commercials in which a big laboratory tells us how wonderful their medicine is but right before the commercial is over, the actor lets us know about all the side effects caused by this wonder drug; things like constipation, dry mouth, vomiting, dizziness, diarrhea etc. Perhaps you have heard about this pill that claims to grow hair in a very small number of people. This drug also causes some undesirable sex malfunctions. Or perhaps you know how a laxative works by irritating the walls of the colon thus giving you the runs.

If you do not agree with the theory that you need to cause small harm to one part of the body to heal another, then you will find this pages very useful.

All the ailments listed here are treated with natural herbs, vitamins, foods, and minerals. That's right, we use only mother nature's tools to cure ourselves, the way it was intended from the beginning of time. This does not mean that we are against modern medicine. We believe that in the past few years this technique has advanced a great deal and many drugs and treatments are necessary to improve our lives. We are against the "business" that makes people believe that the body needs help from chemicals in the form of drugs for every little illness.

A good example would be a common cold. We start sneezing, our nose runs, we cough, we get a fever, all signs that the body is healing itself. Our sneeze is used by the body to expel some strange invader trying to get inside of our respiratory system. Our nose creates mucus to traps particles so that when we blow our nose, the particles are ejected. Fever is the way the body elevates its temperature to kill a harmful virus that has made it inside.

So we go out and buy some medicines to get rid of these symptoms and suppress our immune system. We take them and we feel a little better but it takes the body a lot longer to heal itself. You see what these drugs do is target the symptoms. Sure symptoms are uncomfortable but that's what the body does to heal itself.

Using natural remedies we boost our immune system giving our body the tools and power to heal faster.

We are giving knowledge so that you can see your body like it is, the most perfect machine ever invented, capable of fixing itself if we give it the chance. Even when we treat our bodies badly by smoking, eating the wrong things, drinking etc., the body is always trying to repair what's broken, from a bone to a simple cold.

We would like to thank you, for buying the "Home Made Medicine Book" Third Edition hope that you find many uses for this book to better your health and your family's. By investing in this information you are showing those around you that you care. You care about the well being of your loved ones and you are also making a strong point that you do not want to load yours or your children's bodies with synthetic drugs or harsh chemicals unless is absolutely necessary.

For that, we congratulate you, and we welcome you to a club that is rapidly growing as people around the world take control of their bodies and their health. We are going back to basics, the way it was, the way it was meant to be. You are a mature intelligent individual that has learned that most synthetic drugs cause dangerous and undesirable side effects. You will not be fooled by slick advertising campaigns enticing you to buy their chemical fill products. For all that we applaud you.

Throughout this book you will read things that will shock you, you will learn things that will amaze you and you will make remedies and products that will make you proud. All the knowledge you will gather will make you and your family healthier and don't be surprised if friends come to you for advice. Armed with this book you will have the power to change things for the better while enjoying the peace of mind which comes from knowing that whatever you make is good for you and others. When you decide to start your own garden and make your own remedies and products you will cherish your new hobby. It will give you a chance to relax while you save money.

So, go ahead and start reading. Start making your own products and remedies and see the difference it can make in your life. The book will be here in your computer ready to give you step by step instructions on how to prepare, store, and use herbal preparations. Don't forget to pay extra attention to the areas in the book marked as TIPs they are a fountain of secrets, tips, statistics and amazing information.

Should you have any questions, remember that you can contact me using my web site at www.Charles-Silverman.com thank you again for reading my book.

Charles Silverman N.D. & Staff
www.Charles-Silverman.com

About

Charles Silverman N.D., a Naturalist and Herbalist since 1979, is the author of the HomeMade Medicine book and the www.HomeMadeMedicine.com Web site. Charles lives in Miami, FL and has dedicated a major part of his life to the preparation of natural remedies and natural products to help people with allergies and chemical intolerance. He has traveled around the world from Canada, Germany, France, and India to the mountains of Peru and Argentina (South America) researching and studying the different domestic species of herbs and plants. His articles are published on several web sites like ezinearticles.com and naturalhealthweb.com and he is regularly interviewed by various publications and newspapers like the Montgomery News of Alabama. All his knowledge has been transferred to his web site and now to this amazing book, that takes advantage of the latest technology in order to bring you the most complete guide for home healing ever made.

Be curious always! For knowledge will not acquire you: you must acquire it.

~ Sudie Back ~

The Body as a whole.

TIP: **An estimated 100,000 people are hospitalized and 16,000 die from side effects caused by arthritis drugs alone each year.**

This is a sad but true statistic.

The body becomes ill when a chain of events that develops somewhere in the body ends. The organ where this chain reaction begins may not be the organ where it ends. In other words you may feel a headache but that may not be where the problem is, it could be caused by improper liver function, indigestion, constipation or even by a nerve in your spinal cord. Treating the headache may get rid of the pain but it does not address the real problem.

The body should be treated as a whole. After all, every organ, extremity, even hair is connected to a tissue which is part of the same body. If this makes sense to you then you will agree that a natural holistic healing, using natural home remedies that returns the whole body to a normal balance is the way to treat any illness.

With this book you are in controls of the most complete guide to natural healing, from broken bones, pregnancy problems, remedies children, adults, remedies for skin conditions, to a simple cold. The list is so long that is not practical to mention everything here.

We all agree that personal alternative medicine is becoming one of the most popular methods to treat many diseases. That's why I created this book to bring you an alternative method to heal using herbal medicines.

In our member's area at www.Charles-Silverman.com you will find a remedy and many special herbal preparations for every condition you can imagine, including our revolutionary acne home remedy, this home remedy for acne, provides unbelievable results; it is part of our home remedy library. This is just one example visit my site to learn more.

Natural Home Remedies for a strong Immune System.

Sixty five years ago medical scientists promised us that infections caused by bacteria and others would be a thing of the past due to the new discovery of patented pharmaceutical drugs. This very brave statement was made and almost automatically more than half of the herbs recommended in the U.S. Pharmacopoeia were taken off to be replaced with these chemical drugs. I wish I could tell you that the promised was kept and that now we live in an infection free world, but this is not so. We are all familiar with the enormous amounts and resistance of bacteria. Antibiotics have not live up to their promised; to the contrary they have become a problem in itself, by over use and side effects that cause liver, kidney, nervous and immune system damage.

Modern conventional medicine battles diseases directly by means of drugs, surgery, radiation and other therapies, but true health can be attained only by maintaining a healthy properly functioning immune system and using home remedies can definitely help to strengthen the ability to fight diseases.

It is the immune system that fights off disease-causing microorganisms and it engineers the healing process. The immune system is the key to fighting every kind of insult to the body, from that little shaving scratch to the gigantic amount of viruses the constantly try to invade our bodies. Even the aging process may be related to a deteriorated immune system.

Weakening of the immune system makes us vulnerable to every type of illness that affects humans. Some common signs of impaired immune functions include fatigue, lassitude, repeated infections, inflammation, allergic reactions, slow wound healing, chronic diarrhea and infections related to overgrowth of benign organisms already present in the body, such as oral thrush, vaginal yeast infections and other fungal infections. It is calculated that a normal adult gets an average of two colds per year. People suffering from colds more than the average are likely to have some sort of immune deficiency. Dark circles could be directly related to an immune system malfunction.

Explaining what the immune system is the hard part. The immune system it is not an organ but an interaction between many organs, structures and substances with the task of recognizing or differencing from things that belong and those that don't belong to the body, and then neutralizing or destroying the ones that are foreign.

The immune system is like no other bodily system, the patrolling and protecting tasks of the immune system are share by white cells, bone marrow, the lymphatic vessels and organs, specialized cells found and various body tissues, and specialized substances, called serum factors, that are present in the blood. Ideally, all of these components work together to protects the body against diseases.

To boost and protect your immune system I recommend a list of herbs, vitamins, supplements and special home remedies recipes that have shown remarkable results throughout the years.

Home Remedies to strengthen the immune system.

Home Remedy #1: Astragalus boosts the immune system and generates anticancer cells in the body. It is also a powerful antioxidant and protects the liver from toxins. This makes this plant ideal for people suffering from dark circles due to liver problems and depressed immune system. IMPORTANT: Do not take this herb if fever is present.

Home Remedy #2: Baybarry has antibiotic effects for sore throat, coughs, clods and flu.

Home Remedy #3: Garlic is effective against at least 30 types of bacteria, viruses, parasites and fungi. It has anti-inflammatory and astringent properties.

Home Remedy #4: Echinacea boosts the immune system and enhances lymphatic function.

Home Remedy #5: Goldenseal strengthens the immune system, cleanses and detoxifies the body. It has anti bacteria properties.

Home Remedy #6: In a small town called Chirchik, Russia, a flu epidemic swept the town. When many adults and children did not get sick scientists wanted to know why they were immune to the disease. It turns out that all of them used the berries from an herb called Shizandra.

Home Remedy #7: Include in the diet chlorella, garlic and pearl barley. These foods contain germanium, a trace element beneficial for the immune system. Also giant red kelp contains iodine, calcium, iron, carotene, protein, riboflavin and vitamin C, which are necessary for the immune system's functional integrity.

Home Remedy #8: Vitamin C may be the single most important nutrient for the immune system. It is essential for the formation of adrenal hormones and the production of lymphocytes. It also has direct effect on bacteria and viruses. Vitamin C should be taken with bioflavonoids, natural plant substances that enhance absorption and reinforce the action of this vitamin.

Differents Ways to Prepare Herbs

There are different ways in which herbal remedies can be prepared and many methods are available in all health stores. There are thousands of herbs and almost all parts of the plant can be used for health or healing. They can also be combined to obtain different results. Preparing your own herbal remedies will help you save money and the process of preparing herbs is not complex but if not done properly can result in an ineffective preparation.

Herbs can be prepared to be used internally or externally depending on the nature of the ailment and on the herb itself. Some herbs are more effective when used externally while others act better when used internally. Following you'll find a description of the different ways available to prepare herbs. Later in our book you'll learn how to make, use, and prepare each method for every ailment shown.

Internal use herbal preparations:

GLYCERITES

Some preparations are made with a base of alcohol to extract the ingredients. Glycerites are thick liquids that are alcohol free and utilize glycerin instead of alcohol. This is a great way of treating children because glycerites are sweet making it easy for the parent to introduce them to the child. Also, glycerites do not affect blood sugar levels making them perfect for people with diabetes.

Glycerin is used in our daily life. Foods like frosting and baked goods contain glycerin. It can be obtained from pharmacies.

An average dose of glycerites is about 25 to 30 drops. They are not as potent as tinctures but they should be diluted in water or juices. Using them directly can irritate the mouth. To make a glycerite use the following:

1 ounce of herbs.
6 ounces glycerin.
4 ounce distilled water.

Chop herbs in a blender and place them in a dark glass jar. Mix the glycerin and water and add it to the herbs then close the jar tightly and store at room temperature for 2 weeks. Do not use until then. Shake container every day to move ingredients around. Strain the herb pulp and store in a cool and dark place. A glycerite can last for 2 years.

PILLS

If you have no problems using pills, capsules or tablets you could take advantage of the easiest way of taking herbs especially those that are bitter or spicy. The herb is dried, powdered, processed and either compressed into a pill or placed in capsules made of gelatin. The pills and capsules dissolve in the stomach releasing the ingredients into the bloodstream. Empty capsules can be obtained from health stores so you can combine your own herbs if you can't get the mixture you are looking for.
A pill, capsule or tablet is the equivalent of half cup of tea.

SYRUPS

A syrup is a tincture, liquid extract, glycerite or even a tea with enough honey, glycerin, fruit syrup or molasses to thicken its consistency. Since they contain sugar, syrups can be a problem for people suffering from diabetes. Children under two years of age can not eat honey. A syrup makes a great remedy for sore throat, cough, colds or flu. It coats the membranes soothing and protecting them. To make a syrup formula use the following:

6 tbs.. of herbs.
1 pint of water.
4 ounces of glycerin.
1 ounce fruit syrup or honey (don't use honey for children under 2 years of age).

Boil herbs and water, remove from heat and steep for 45 minutes. Filter and place the liquid on the stove again, simmer for 10 minutes and remove from heat. Take one cup of liquid and add glycerin and fruit syrup or honey while the liquid still hot. Stored in the refrigerator, it will last for 6 months.

TEAS

Teas are the easiest and cheapest way of preparing herbs. Some herbs act better and quicker when taken with hot water. The only drawback to drinking tea is that some herbs really taste bad. It only costs a few cents per dose and some herb combinations provide fast relief.
There are two different ways to prepare a tea:

Infusions are made by pouring hot or boiling water on the herbs and steeping for a period of time, usually 20 to 45 minutes. Commercially prepared tea bags are ground fine to make tea faster usually in about 5 minutes.

Cold infusions are made by placing herbs in cold water and letting them sit for about 8 hours. This method is used when the herbs are sensitive to heat or lose their essential oils when heated.

DECOCTIONS

Whenever the herb to be used is hard and woody it is better to make a decoction rather than an infusion or tea, to ensure that the soluble contents of the herbs actually reach the water. Since many herb preparations consist of using bark, roots, wood, nuts and seeds, it is necessary to boil the herb. More heat has to be used in order to get through the hard and strong walls of these herbs.

Decoctions are prepared by simmering the herbs for 30 minutes or longer. The high temperature over a long period of time releases more properties from thick barks and roots. Remember to keep the heat low and cover the saucepan in order to keep the essential properties inside and to avoid too much evaporation.

If the recipe you are making calls for the use of soft and hard herbs, I recommend you make a decoction and an infusion separately, then combine the two liquids. This way the sensitive properties of the soft herb remain intact and the hard to get properties from the hard herb is collected as well. However, if the hard herb contains oil, it is best to powder it and then use in an infusion rather than a decoction to ensure that the volatile oil does not evaporate.

To prepare a decoction follow the step below.

1.- Put one tsp. of dried herb (broken into small pieces) or three tsp. of fresh herb (cut into small pieces) in a saucepan and add one cup of water. These are general proportions.

2.- Boil and simmer for about 30 minutes or the time given for the mixture you are preparing. If the herb contains some oils, put a lid on the saucepan to avoid evaporation.

3.- Strain the herbs while the preparation is still hot.

TINCTURES

Tinctures are also called liquid extracts and are the most potent herb preparation due to the concentration of the herbal medicine. Tinctures can be used externally as an antiseptic, disinfectant or local antibiotic. This concentrated form of herbs is very useful for people who are taking large doses of a bad tasting herb. Since the strength of tinctures is very high they should be taken in a diluted form mixed with juices.

Tinctures are made with alcohol to extract the properties and compound in the herbs to make them more powerful and faster acting. Even though we are talking about a very potent herb preparation the dosage can be estimated. These are herbs that are very safe even for a child. There is no danger of poisoning unlike synthetic drugs that can be fatal. To prepare a tincture you mix:

1 ounce of dried or powdered herbs.
5 ounces of vodka (vodka is 50 % alcohol).

Chop herbs in a blender and put them in a dark glass jar. Cover the herbs with vodka making sure they are completely submerged. Close jar tightly and store in a dark, dry and cool place for 2 weeks at room temperature. Shake the jar every day enough to move the herbs and liquid around. After 2 weeks filter the herb pulp and store in a cool place. A tincture can last for more then 5 years.

VINEGARS

The process of making herbal vinegar is similar to the one used to prepare tinctures but in the first one vinegar is used to get the properties of the herb instead of alcohol. Vinegar herbs are not as potent as tincture but they do not contain alcohol and they can be used in meals such as salads which makes them easy to take.

TIP: Vinegar damages tooth enamel so make sure you rinse your mouth with water after drinking it. To make a vinegar formula use the following:

1 ounce fresh or dried herbs.
5 ounces vinegar (any kind).

Chop herbs in a blender and put them in a dark glass jar. Cover the herbs with vinegar making sure they are completely submerged. Close jar tightly and store in a dark, dry and cool place for 2 weeks at room temperature. Shake the jar every day enough to move the herbs and liquid around. After 2 weeks filter the herb pulp and store in a cool place. A tincture can last for more then 2 years.

External use herbal preparations:

BODY OILS

Body oils are made from essential oils and are used for massage of injuries such as muscles, burns, bruises etc. They are a good alternative for children who refuse to take herbs orally. Body oils are also used for skin conditions and skin care, especially facial treatments, although they take longer to act, they are a good supplement to other remedies.

COMPRESS

A compress is made by soaking a towel, cotton cloth, or cotton in a strong herbal tea, tincture, essential oil or glycerites and then placed on the skin. Is a great way to treat headaches, muscle injuries, burns, infections, fibroids, bruises, sore throats and any other condition that requires increased circulation to the affected area.

HERBAL BATH

Herbal baths are a good way to treat stress related ailments. Aromatherapy is very popular and uses herbs to induce relaxation and distention. We all know that stress is one of the most common disease causing conditions. Placing herbs and oils in the bath can help control brain activity. I'm sure this has happened to you at least once, you are walking and all of the sudden you smell a perfume and almost immediately memories come rushing back: memories of a person or a situation or a place. That's the principal behind herbal baths and aromatherapy. Herbal baths can also be used to cure foot problems or nail infections and many skin conditions as well.

POULTICE

A poultice is made by placing herbs on the injured area. The most effective way of making a poultice is by grinding or blending the herbs to a fine powder. Sometimes the final result is a sticky paste that can be spread on the skin. If the herbs are too dried a few drops of water added can help obtain the desired consistency. To make a stronger poultice tinctures, glycerates or essential oils can be used instead of water. A poultice can also be wrapped in order to keep heat or moisture in. To make a poultice use the following:

1 handful of herbs.
4 ounces of water.

Blend all ingredients until the consistency resembles a thick slurry. Place the poultice on the affected area and wrap with a gauze. Keep it in place for one hour. A poultice can be placed in an ice cube tray and frozen. Store the cubes in a plastic bag and thaw when needed.

SALVE or OINTMENT

A salve is a herbal oil but thicker. It is very useful in cases of cuts, scrapes, rashes, swelling, infections, poison ivy and poison oak or any skin condition with the exception of burns. It's recommended not to use oily substances on burns because It keeps the heat In and causes more pain. A very popular salve is olive oil which has many healing properties.

To make a salve or ointment follow the steps below:

1.- Make 500 ml/ 1 pt. of infusion or decoction extract.

2.- Place in a saucepan 2 oz./ 60 gr. of White wax, 3 oz./ 90 gr. of Lard (pig's solid fat) and 3 oz./ 90 ml. of Almond oil.

3.- Add the 500 ml. of tea from step 1.- and stir.

4.- Simmer until the water from the tea has evaporated completely. Make sure not to over heat. If desired, you can use a bigger pan with

2 inches of water and then place the smaller pan containing the ingredients inside of the first one to avoid burning.

5.- Add 3 drops of benzoin tincture.

6.- Place the mixture in a container with a tight lid.

DRYING and STORING HERBS and ROOTS

Herbs should be dried by spreading them in loose, single layers on a flat surface or on a wire rack similar to the ones used in your oven. This allows air to get underneath the plant and to ensure an even and quicker drying. If you are using a flat surface to dry herbs make sure to turn them frequently. To dry herbs follow these steps.

1.- Harvest the exposed part of the plant, leaves and stems by cutting with a sharp knife or scissors. Make sure not to tear the plant as this can cause it to stop growing or die.

2.- Strip the leaves and flowers from the main stem.

3.- Spread out on the rack and place in the sun or in a warm dry place until they are brittle and crumble easily.

4.- Pack them in Zip Lock bags or dark glass containers with a tight lid and keep them away from sun light or heat.

Roots are perhaps the most difficult part of a plant to dry because they are thick and very moist. Removing a root from the ground can be very messy, depending on the type of plant being removed. Some herbs have roots that spread over a wide area. Once the root is out it must be washed to remove excess soil and placed in shelves for about 10 days. Roots lose 75% of their weight in drying.

1.- Remove root from the ground. Wash root to remove dirt.

2.- Cut off the top part and rootlets. Chop the root in slices 2 inches long (if the root is big). This will make them dry faster.

3.- Spread out on a rack in a warm, dry place for 10 days. Store in a oven or other dry and warm place for 10 more days.

Antioxidants.

Many of the studies and research done lately has focused on the nutrients known as antioxidants.
Scientists are beginning to understand the preventive qualities of antioxidants but the average person does not yet understand what antioxidants do or what they are. But you will have that knowledge after reading this section.

Understanding the function of antioxidants is not hard and taking advantage of their properties is quite simple. Diseases like Cancer and arteriosclerosis are unable to advance and spread through the body thanks to the actions of antioxidants like Vitamin C, A, E, Beta-carotene and others. By blocking and neutralizing the destructive power of too many free radicals, these antioxidants allow us to prevent major diseases. A clear example of this is the remarkable reduction of breast cancer in women who consume raw and cocked spinach and carrots.

Why are they called antioxidant?

Latest research has shown scientists that oxygen, the gas we depend on to live, creates some very harmful by-products that destroy the very life it helps sustain. There are several vitamins that reverse or slow the oxidation cause by oxygen. That is the reason they call them antioxidants.
Oxidation, the reaction of oxygen with other chemicals, is the process that causes metals to rust, wood to burn, and a sliced apple to turn brown. As a matter of fact, if you coat a sliced apple with an antioxidant such as vitamin C, the apple will take a lot longer to change color.

It is best to remember that vitamin and mineral supplements should never be used as substitutes for a healthy, well balanced diet! It is also important to note that we can "over- supplement" our bodies by taking much more than the recommended daily value of certain vitamins and minerals.

Vitamins A and E are fat soluble, meaning that excess amounts are stored in the liver and fatty tissues, instead of being quickly excreted, creating a risk of toxicity and disease. Your best bet is to eat a diet rich in fruits, veggies, and whole grains. Sweet potatoes, carrots, spinach, cantaloupe and mangoes are great sources of antioxidants.

A healthy level of free radicals is needed by the body in order to get rid of bacteria. Free radicals are atoms or groups of atoms that have at least one unpaired electron, which makes them highly reactive. Free radicals promote beneficial oxidation that produces energy and kills bacterial invaders. In excess, however, they produce harmful oxidation that can damage cell membranes and cell contents.

It is known that people who eat adequate amounts of fruits and vegetables high in antioxidants have a lower incidence of cardiovascular disease, certain cancers, and cataracts. Fruits and vegetables are rich in antioxidants but it is not known which dietary factors are responsible for the beneficial effects. Each plant contains hundreds of phytochemicals (plant chemicals) whose presence is dictated by hereditary factors. Only well-designed long-term research can determine whether any of these chemicals, taken in a pill, would be useful for preventing any disease.

Without a doubt antioxidants are a vital tool in our fight against diseases. We all agree that sometimes eating the right thing is difficult but when compared with pain and suffering that we can bring to ourselves by getting cancer, arthritis or arteriosclerosis, a bowl of salad and an orange seems like a very tasty choice.

In this book you will find a remedy and many special herbal preparations for every condition you can imagine. We all agree that personal alternative medicine is becoming one of the most popular treatments for many diseases.

Researchers Identify the 20 Most Antioxidant-Rich Foods
1. Red beans
2. Wild blueberries
3. Red kidney beans
4. Pinto beans
5. Cultivated blueberries
6. Cranberries

7. Artichokes
8. Blackberries
9. Prunes
10. Raspberries
11. Strawberries
12. Red delicious apples
13. Granny Smith apples
14. Pecans
15. Sweet cherries
16. Black plums
17. Russet potatoes
18. Black beans
19. Plums
20. Gala apples

4 Ways In Which You Can Use Coenzyme Q10.

Sometimes I ask myself why this wonderful antioxidant supplement was given such a technical name, many people feel intimidated by the name alone, thus refusing to take CoQ10. But the truth is that this nutrient is one of the most effective antioxidants and it has been proven to help many serious diseases. We will study in depth the benefits and properties that researchers have found in this "vitamin like" substance called Coenzyme Q10. Probably you haven't even heard the name Coenzyme Q10, or if you have, you don't even know what it does or why you should take it. The potential and most of the properties found in CoQ10 have been recognized rather recently. CoQ10 is known to scientists as ubiquinol. This is a naturally occurring nutrient normally present in every cell in the body so it is only logical to believe that it plays an important part in treating and preventing many conditions. The body makes CoQ10, but most likely the majority of people don't make it well or enough of it. The good news is that we can absorb CoQ10 from foods, especially fish, and meats (particularly organ meats like liver, kidney, etc., more on this later), the bad news is that most people don't eat these types of meats, plus as we age the body loses it efficiency in manufacturing important nutrients. It has been proven that people suffering from heart diseases and cancer have lower levels of CoQ10, thus supplementation is recommended.

1. CoQ10 helps in the energy production within each cell

The body, just like a car, needs fuel. Our primary source of fuel is through fats, proteins, and carbohydrates in our diet. After digestion in the stomach, the nutrients from foodstuffs are absorbed into the bloodstream and circulate to various tissues and cells. The cells have to break down the sugars, fats and amino acids in a form that makes energy. This energy production occurs in organelles, or microscopic organ-like structures, called mitochondria, and CoQ10 plays a key role in this activity.

There are hundreds, sometimes thousands, of mitochondria within each cell. In a sense, they are the factories of your cells, with the final product being energy. The energy that is produced is stored in a chemical called adenosine triphosphate, or simply ATP. It is carried by electrons and protons which are sub atomic particles. These energetic electrons and protons are moved around in cells to their destinations by numerous compounds. CoQ10 is one of the most important compounds.

2. CoQ10 as an antioxidant

CoQ10 also serves as an antioxidant, which is its second role. By controlling the movement of electrons, CoQ10 limits the production of dangerous free radicals, which are molecules lacking one electron in what should be a pair. To learn more about free radicals and antioxidants go here http://www.homemademedicine.com/articles/antioxidants.html

So far many researches and clinical studies have shown CoQ10 to be an amazing tool that helps us fight and prevent many dangerous conditions. Among these are:

Congestive heart failure
Coronary artery disease
High cholesterol
High blood pressure
Mitral valve prolapse
Breast Cancer
Periodontitis or Gingivitis
and Fatigue

3. CoQ10 prevents many conditions

Another important aspect in the uses of CoQ10, is the prevention of many conditions, CoQ10 helps maintain normal heart function and preventing serious heart disease. Our heart works 24 hrs a day, using lots of energy, to pump blood though the body, and since CoQ10 plays an important role in energy production, it has shown to be a very valuable heart energizing nutrient.

But why doctors don't recommend more the use of CoQ10?

Hundreds of scientific studies have been published on CoQ10, including many involving humans. CoQ10 has also been the subject of ten international scientific and medical meetings. Furthermore, the role of CoQ10 in energy production was basis of the 1978 Nobel prize in chemistry, given to Peter Mitchell, Ph.D.

Unfortunately, most doctors in the US are not familiar with the published research regarding the potential of CoQ10 because many of the journals they read rarely discuss the benefits of this and many other nutrients. The reason for this is very simple, nutrients cannot be patented so they are of very little interest to pharmaceutical companies and drug manufacturing laboratories and these are the companies that sponsor and publish most of the journals read by doctors. However, traveling around Europe, China, Japan and South America, has shown me that the story is completely different in the rest of the world, where most health-care professionals are treating their patients with heart failure and other conditions by prescribing CoQ10. In fact, CoQ10 is the fifth most commonly prescribed "drug" in Japan.

4. How to get it from food

How much CoQ10 do we get from foods and is it enough?

Dietary intake of CoQ10 normally ranges from 2 to 20 mg a day. Most of this comes from meats and fish. The richest source of CoQ10 is organ meat, like liver, kidney, and heart. If you don't eat these types of meats, chances are that your body does not have adequate level of CoQ10. Supplements in these cases is recommended. Younger people tend to get enough CoQ10 from food and from their own body production, but as we age the ability of the body to make and absorb CoQ10 drops significantly. For people in the middle age group, I recommend a dosage of 30mg a day, although people taking 60 to 100 mg a day have reported a significant improvement in alertness, energy level, motivation, mood elevation, and enhanced focus. Fortunately, CoQ10 has no serious side effects. Only 1.5 percent of people taking 60 to 100 mg a day have reported nausea and insomnia due to the energizing effects of CoQ10. Also, this wonderful nutrient can be taken for years non-stop with only positive results. I recommend to start slow, with a dosage of 10 mg a day and gradually increase it to the desired dosage or until satisfactory results have been achieved.

I hope this information helps you come to the conclusion that Coenzyme Q10 is one of most important essential nutrients which is needed for a healthy body and to treat several conditions.

Vitamin A

Vitamin A comes from animal sources such as eggs and meat and is present in the form of a precursor called beta-carotene, when manufactured by plants.

Vitamin A is found in milk, cheese, cream, liver, kidney, cod and halibut fish oil. All of these sources, except for skim milk that has been fortified with vitamin A, are high in saturated fat and cholesterol. The vegetable sources of beta-carotene are fat and cholesterol free. The body regulates the conversion of beta-carotene to vitamin A based on the body's needs. Sources of beta-carotene are carrots, pumpkin, sweet potatoes, winter squashes, cantaloupe, pink grapefruit, apricots, broccoli, spinach, and most dark green, leafy vegetables. The more intense the color of a fruit or vegetable, the higher the beta-carotene content.

Functions

Vitamin A helps in the formation and maintenance of healthy teeth, skeletal and soft tissue, mucous membranes, and skin. It is also known as retinol, as it generates the pigments that are necessary for the working of the retina. It promotes good vision, especially in dim light. It may also be required for reproduction and lactation. Beta carotene, which has antioxidant properties, is a precursor to vitamin A.

Recommendations

Recommended daily allowances (RDAs) are defined as the levels of intake of essential nutrients that the Food and Nutrition Board judges to be adequate to meet the known nutrient needs of almost all healthy persons.

The best way to get the daily requirement of essential vitamins is to eat a balanced diet that contains a variety of foods from the food guide pyramid.

Side Effects

Vitamin A deficiency can increase the susceptibility to infectious diseases, as well as cause vision problems. When you are seriously deficient in vitamin A, your body suffers dire consequences: your bones, reproductive organs, skin, and your respiratory tract all begin to malfunction.

Large doses of vitamin A can be toxic, although you would have to take about 50,000 IU or more daily for an extended period of time, that's ten times the RDA for you to develop signs of intoxication. Vitamin A overdose can also cause abnormal fetal development in pregnant women. Increased amounts of beta-carotene can turn the color of skin to yellow or orange. The skin color returns to normal once the increased intake of beta-carotene is reduced.

We recommend taking beta-carotene instead of vitamin A, since beta-carotene is not toxic even in large amounts, because the body takes only the amount needed and converts that into vitamin A while the rest is excreted.

Garlic Food or Medicine

Are you worried about your health? Are you anxious about your heart or about the possibility of contracting cancer? If so, you are not alone and your concerns are quite valid. Cancer and heart disease are today's major killers, and as of now, we are yet to find a safe and effective drug that can prevent these diseases. Some will argue that taking one or two aspirins a day can reduce the risk of heart disease, and it saddens me to see how many people are doing this, because I know the problems brought on by aspirin over use. If these people knew about the long term damage caused by this drug, they would think twice before popping another one into their mouths. Maybe they would give up that harmful habit if they learn that there is a better answer to preventing these and other diseases. What is the answer? The herb called Garlic. But don't just take my word; even scientists are supporting its properties.

A lot of people use garlic in cooking without knowing that this herb has quite a few medicinal uses. Although Garlic has been around for several thousands of years, its origins are quite obscure. It is thought to have come from Russia making its way to the Mediterranean countries. Garlic was known to be used in the diets of ancient Egyptians, Romans, and Greeks.

Garlic is known to aid digestion, ward off colds, infection, expel worms, ease chest congestion, help alleviate rheumatism and cleanse the intestines. In World War I, garlic juice was used on the sterile bandages to prevent infection. Garlic has also been known to help hardening of the arteries, sinus problems, skin complexion, and hay fever if taken in capsule form on a regular basis.

This herb has been studied, and the results are amazing. Garlic contains a large number of sulphur compounds. One of these compounds is diallyl disulphide which has remarkable anti-cancer properties. This compound prevents two early stages of carcinogenesis, initiation and promotion, from developing. The anti-initiator activity is the result of two complementary mechanisms:

- diallyl disulphide prevents certain carcinogenic substances from being activated

- moreover, this molecule stimulates enzymes capable of neutralising the activity of carcinogenic substances

These two mechanisms reduce the toxicity of carcinogens to cell DNA. Diallyl disulphide is metabolised in the liver into an oxide compound that may be behind the effects described.

In both cases, these studies have dealt with cancer prevention in rat liver, but the mechanisms brought to light give reason to believe that their scope is much wider: effects on other cancers, potential extrapolation to humans.

As fruit and vegetables are rich in minor constituents, nutritionists have increasingly shown an interest in their role in the prevention of cancers, cardiovascular diseases and inflammatory diseases over the last decade.

One the most interesting stories of the properties of garlic, came to me from South Africa, Professor Sid Cywes, a former paediatric surgeon at University of Cape Town was having trouble hybridizing his orchids seeds. The trouble was a fungal infection in his culture medium. Mr Peter De Wet, a chief research technologist and Prof Cywes hatched a plan that entailed a dose of garlic. To their astonishment administering garlic to their orchid culture medium killed the mould. They then went on to test garlic's ability to combat the yeast Candida. At that time one of Prof. Cywe's patients, a baby at the Red Cross Hospital had a serious Candida infection down the entire length of its oesophagus and gastro-intestinal tract. A garlic solution added to the baby's milk cured the child within 48 hours.

Since then about thirty very sick infants, where broad spectrum antibiotics failed to bring improvement, have been given fresh allicin enterally. The allicin treatment brought about a significant success. However, this was not a controlled clinical study.

One of the active ingredients in garlic is a compound called allicin. On crushing fresh garlic, an enzyme called alliinase is released which rapidly converts the odorless compound alliin into allicin bearing the typical odor of garlic. Allicin is highly unstable and rapidly converts to other sulfur-compounds such as ajoene. It is, however, allicin and ajoene which have been the main subject of research. These compounds block the enzymes which are necessary for metabolism of the micro-organisms. They have been shown to inhibit the growth of more than 23 organisms. A very interesting point is that no resistance to allicin has been found up to date.

Garlic supplements are one of the best ways to get the daily intake of its properties and compounds, without the breath issue. When combined with vitamin E, garlic becomes a powerful antioxidant as well.

Garlic and its compounds, have been tested against the bacteria Helicobacter pylori and it had tremendous success. Allicin has also been shown to inhibit Campylobacter- universally recognized as the most common cause of gastro-enteritis in very young children of low-income families. These findings are of much interest as bacteria including Helicobacter and Campylobacter are becoming increasingly resistant to antibiotics.

I just hope that more people are exposed to this information so they can make a wiser decision when it comes to preventing diseases like the ones we discussed here. Please send this article to your friends and loved ones, share with them the information you have, help them keep their health.

The Facts about Green tea.

Do you drink Green Tea?

Lately, green tea has been getting a lot of attention. Recent reports and scientific studies found that green tea has the ability to greatly reduce the risk of many cancers and in some cases it has shown signs of reducing tumors. However, green tea has been around for thousands of years. In China and Japan it is used as a tonic that keeps the body in optimum conditions.

We will dive into the secrets and properties and we will study green tea to expose all of its properties. We will answer questions like what makes some teas cure illnesses and what is the difference between a regular black tea and this wonderful green healing concoction.

Chances are you have already tasted green tea. It is a common treat in most Asian restaurants. What you probably did not realize is that you were drinking a powerful healing remedy. Green tea has been used for more than 4,000 years for medicinal purposes. Only recently are scientists paying attention to this marvelous plant. As we mentioned green tea can prevent cancer but that is not all. Other research has shown that green tea bolsters the heart's resistance to cardiovascular diseases, increases longevity, detoxifies the body and boosts the immune system.

TIP: Green tea also prevents cavities.

Why does green tea have all these properties and black tea doesn't?

Although green and black tea come from the same plant, it is the processing that sets them apart. Tea leaves contain an enzyme that causes the leaves to oxidate after picking. By steaming and heating the leaves, processors are able to stop the oxidation process. Black tea is left to oxidate and it is submitted to several more possessing steps which causes it to turn dark brown and sometimes red.

Unfortunately, this manipulation of the plant reduces and destroys compounds called polyphenols present in the freshly picked leaves. These compounds are the secret healing weapon contained in the green tea leaves. Because it is processed as little as possible, green tea retains all its polyphenols. Out of all the types of teas, green tea contains the highest levels of polyphenols.

What are polyphenols and what do they do?

Polyphenols are a group of natural phytochemicals (plant chemicals). These phytochemicals are potent antioxidants and antioxidants are the substances that protect the body from free radicals and free radicals are the reactive molecules that damage the body at the cellular level causing cancer, heart disease and many other horrible diseases. (To learn more about antioxidants and free radicals read Antioxidants).

There are primarily four types of antioxidants in green tea that stand out and which give it the properties for which green tea is famous. Many other nutrients can be found in green tea. Vitamin C tops the list. Green tea contains ten times more vitamin C than black tea. Also found in different levels are vitamin B2, vitamin D, vitamin K and carotenoids (beta-carotine).

The wrong information gives bad reputation.

Many years ago there were concerns raised which made people believe that drinking tea in general might interfere with the body's absorption and use of iron which in turns causes anemia. Further research has determined that tea does not increase the risk of iron-deficiency anemia.

Another concern that was raised was the seemingly high level of mineral aluminum sometimes found in tea. Aluminum causes bone and brain disorders. Again further research shows that the type of aluminum found in tea does not react in any harmful way in the body.

As far as we know, for thousands of years tea has been used without any adverse reaction or downside.

Green tea and cancer prevention

As mentioned before, green tea has a 4,000 year old reputation as a health enhancing beverage. Although this reputation has been dismissed in the past, modern epidemiologists have paid close attention to this plant and they have found proof that many diseases are prevented by drinking green tea.

One of the researches was done in a region of Japan called Shizuoka. They concentrated in that area because statistics showed that both men and women of this city had a way below average rate of death from cancer. A deeper study showed that in this tea growing region, its citizens drank more cups of green tea than the average Japanese citizen.

After this study, dozens more have taken place, some in Europe and some in the United States and the results only fortify the early conclusions. Green tea reduces the risk of cancer.

Ginkgo Biloba

In this section we will talk about one of the oldest and most important herbs, Ginkgo Biloba. After reading the history and benefits of this plant you'll appreciate the true potential of Ginkgo Biloba.

So let's get started !!!

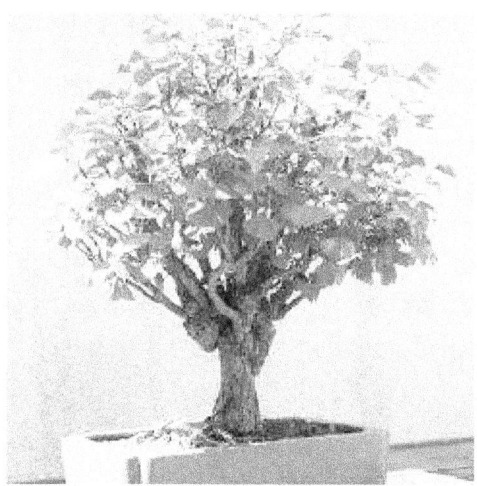

The history

Ginkgo is the oldest living tree, it has seen the rise and fall of dinosaurs, some scientists call it "the living fossil". During the Triassic period it was common in many parts of the world, but it almost vanished completely during the Ice Age, surviving only in Asia. Chinese have used Ginkgo for thousands of years, (as early as 2800 B.C.E.), and it was so important that emperors cultivated the plant as a secret tree within the wall of their temples.

The Properties

Sadly, in America, medicine and health are a big business so the properties of this tree are not publicized. Europeans have come to rely on Ginkgo extract to treat many illnesses. In Germany and France it's been registered as a drug and it's one of the most commonly prescribed remedies. In Germany Ginkgo has been authorized for the treatment of a wide array of cerebral problems, ranging from ringing in the ears, to memory loss, done in Germany and France have shown extremely good results using Ginkgo Biloba extract to treat Alzheimer's, even reversing the disease when caught early.

The main property of Ginkgo is its ability to improve circulation to all parts of the body, including the brain. This is believed to be a key benefit to Alzheimer's and stroke patients. By improving blood flow Ginkgo helps the body deliver essential nutrients and oxygen to damaged areas of the body.

Ginkgo nourishes blood vessels which decreases the chances of heart attacks and circulatory problems.

Another property of Ginkgo is the ability to fight free radicals (see antioxidants). Due to its antioxidant characteristics Ginkgo searches for free radicals, attacking them and leaving harmless molecules in their place.

We need a change

In the United States millions of people have discovered the powerful benefits of Ginkgo biloba and are turning to it for the relief of many conditions related to aging. Thanks to these advocates, Ginkgo has become the third best selling herb in this country. This has raised the attention of big laboratories; realizing the importance of capturing part of this growing market, they are starting to investigate and research this tree, although they have been reluctant to do so because it is almost impossible to patent something that can be grown on anybody's backyard. However, in the future we might see mass-produced herbal remedies manufactured by these big labs and with the complete authorization and support of the FDA.
The good news is that herbs like Ginkgo Biloba will then receive the credit and appreciation they deserve. The bad news is that you should expect a much higher price.

Dosage

Ginkgo Biloba can be taken in capsules, 120-240 mg daily is the recommended amount. If taking a standardized dose, 40 mg 3 times a day should be the proper amount. A tincture can be used and the proper dosage is 10-15 drops 1-3 times a day.

Side effects

Like many herbs, Ginkgo has no dangerous side effects. It is safe during pregnancy or lactation. However, some anticoagulant drugs are not compatible with Ginkgo and it should be avoided if using drugs like warfarin.

Ginseng

At this time we will talk about one of the most popular and controversial herbs, Ginseng. When we say controversial we mean in the United States, in China and Europe there is no controversy about ginseng. This plant has been used for more than 5000 years.

The plant grows in rich woods throughout eastern and central North America, especially along the mountains from Quebec and Ontario, south to Georgia. It was used by the North American Indians. It is a smooth perennial herb with a large, fleshy, very slow-growing root 2 to 3 inches in length (occasionally twice this size) and from ½ to 1 inch in thickness. Its main portion is spindle-shaped and heavily annulated (ringed growth), with a roundish summit, often with a slight terminal projecting point.

At the lower end of this straight portion, there is a narrower continuation, turned obliquely outward in the opposite direction and a very small branch is occasionally borne in the fork between the two. Some small rootlets exist upon the lower portion. The color ranges from a pale yellow to a brownish color. It has a mucilaginous sweetness, approaching that of licorice, accompanied with some degree of bitterness and a slight aromatic warmth, with little or no smell. The stem is simple and erect, about a foot high, bearing three leaves, each divided into five finely-toothed leaflets and a single, terminal umbel, with a few small, yellowish flowers. The fruit is a cluster of bright red berries.

Chinese Ginseng is a larger plant but presents practically the same appearance and habits of growth. Its culture in the United States has never been attempted, though it would appear to be a promising field for experiment.
Panax is not official in the British Pharmacopoeia and it was dismissed from the United States Pharmacopceia at a late revision. It is cultivated almost entirely for export to China.

In China, both varieties are used particularly for dyspepsia, vomiting and nervous disorders. A decoction of 1/2 oz. of the root, boiled in tea or soup and taken every morning, is a commonly held remedy for consumption and other diseases.
In Western medicine it is considered a mild stomachic tonic and stimulant, useful in loss of appetite and in digestive affections that

arise from mental and nervous exhaustion.

A tincture has been prepared from the genuine Chinese or American root, dried and coarsely powdered, covered with five times its weight in alcohol and allowed to stand, well-stoppered, in a dark, cool place, being shaken twice a day. The tincture, poured off and filtered, has a clear, light-lemon color.

The German health authorities allow Asian ginseng products to be labeled as a tonic for invigoration to treat fatigue, reduced work capacity and concentration, and as a tonic during convalescence.

Most reliable clinical studies on Asian ginseng have been conducted in Europe. These studies have generally involved extracts of Asian ginseng standardized to 4 percent and 7 percent of ginsenosides. Results included a shortening of time to react to visual and auditory stimuli, increased respiratory quotient, increased alertness, power of concentration, grasp of abstract concepts, and increases in visual and motor coordination. These are all measures of adaptogenic response.

The vast majority of scientific research, including pharmacological and clinical studies conducted over the past forty years on ginseng has involved Panax ginseng and Chinese ginseng (also called Korean or Asian ginseng). Research has focused on radioprotective, antitumor, antiviral, and metabolic effects; antioxidant activities; nervous system and reproductive performance; effects on cholesterol and lipid metabolism, and endocrinological activity. Research also suggests that ginseng has non-specific immunostimulatory activity similar to that of Echinacea. The active constituents of ginseng are called saponins. According to recent reports, there are at least 18 saponins found in Asian ginseng. American and Asian ginseng both contain different combinations of ginsenosides which can, in part, explain their different activities as understood by Asian traditional medicine practitioners.

CAUTION: Don't take Ginseng and Ginseng mixtures with Coffee as it will accelerate the caffine effects on the body and can cause diarrhea.

Ginseng herb has a long history of use as an alternative medicine going back over 5,000 years and appears on several continents (origin unknown). It is and was used extensively in Native American medicine. The root is adaptogen, cardiotonic, demulcent, panacea, sedative, sialagogue, stimulant, tonic and stomachic. Ginseng has been studied over the past 30 years in many countries, its remarkable ability to help the body adapt to mental and emotional stress, fatigue, heat, cold, and even hunger is confirmed and documented! The major constituents in Ginseng are Triterpenoid saponins, Ginsenosides (at least 29 have been identified), Acetylenic compounds, Panaxans, and Sesquiterpenes. Taken over an extended period it is used to increase mental and physical performance. It is medicinal and therapeutic for the whole body. A very powerful medicinal herb, it both stimulates and relaxes the nervous system, encourages the secretion of hormones, improves stamina, lowers blood sugar and cholesterol levels and increases resistance to disease. The ginsenosides that produce these effects are very similar to the body's own natural stress hormones. It is used in the treatment of debility associated with old age or illness, lack of appetite, insomnia, stress, shock and chronic illness. Ginseng also increases immune function, resistance to infection, and supports liver function. The leaf is emetic and expectorant. The root is candied and used as an edible medicinal kind of candy.

Goldenseal

The Healing Properties of Goldenseal.

Goldenseal has a long history of use as an infection-fighting herb. Now, more than ever, we need safe alternatives to pharmaceutical antibiotics. Most people are unaware of the powerful antimicrobial effects of goldenseal, and the research that supports the use of goldenseal as a natural antibiotic.

Goldenseal is a herb native to eastern North America. Goldenseal is a potent antimicrobial that kills trouble-causing microorganisms, such as bacteria, fungi, and protozoa. It effectively combats a variety of infectious diseases that are often treated with antibiotics but without the harmful side effects of synthetics drugs. If you have any type of bacterial or parasitic infection, goldenseal is probably the best herb you can use. It fights bronchial and sinus infections, strep throat, urinary infections and skin, eye, and gum infections. When used together with echinacea, the pair not only provides the benefits mentioned but also strengthens the immune system and increases the wide range of harmful microorganisms.

Used externally, Goldenseal it is very successful in treating cuts and wounds, boils, and other bacterial skin infections, as well as fungal infections such as athlete's foot and ringworm, eczema, acne and eye infections such as conjunctivitis and hemorrhoids. Internally, goldenseal is used for colds, digestive upsets, and inflamed mucous membranes anywhere in the body. Also helps sore throat and intestinal infections caused by microbes, such as traveler's diarrhea.

Goldenseal is very safe and potent and no dangerous side effects have been reported. However, since one of its characteristic effects is its uterine-stimulating properties, goldenseal should not be used during pregnancy. Some people are allergic to some plants and that is why you should first try goldenseal in a small dose to test for allergic reactions.

Today Goldenseal and herbs in general are back in vogue. The use of herbal and home remedies is no longer regarded as outdated and this means that in the future we might be able to enjoy a more affordable health system as they do in Europe. If you are interested in treating your illnesses in a natural and cost-effective way, then, you need to learn how herbs are mixed and prepared. You need recipes that combine the right herbs in the right amounts.

Echinacea

The immune system may be the most complex system of your body, and scientist are still discovering new information from different studies done on glands, cells and organs that are in charge of keeping the body healthy. It is easy to answer the questions: what does the organ called heart does? Or what do the lungs do? But when it comes to the immune system, not everybody can tell you with exactitude what it is or how it does its job.

Where is the Immune System and what does it do?

The immune system has no specific position in the body, since there are many parts that constitute the immune system and they are spread apart throughout the body. For example the thymus gland located at the base of the neck produces T-cells, the white blood cells in charge of providing us with immunity to known diseases; the spleen, located on the left part of the abdomen, produces general white cells, cleanses the blood of bacteria and destroys old, worn out red blood cells. Then we have the bone marrow and the large network of lymph nodes like the tonsils, located in different parts of the body, but, mainly concentrated in the armpits, neck, groin, abdomen, and chest.

The primary job of the immune system is to protect the body from infectious microorganisms and to prevent the development of cancer. The immune system patrols our body, like a security guard patrolling a mall. The immune system provides two kinds of protections: nonspecific resistance to disease and specific resistance to disease or immunity:

Nonspecific resistance to disease is the first part of the immune system that confronts any microorganism that makes it into the body. These first barriers of defense are; the skin, fever (which kills viruses and bacteria), and inflammation (which causes extra blood to rush to the affected area). The increased number of white blood cells kills the invaders, the mucous membranes, antimicrobial chemicals in our system, and killer cells (which kill tumor cells and infectious microorganisms).

Specific resistance to disease refers to the ability of the body to recognize a previous invader and trigger an immune reaction.

Such a complex system of organs and cells must be kept in balance, otherwise the infection fighting capabilities may decline leaving us exposed and defenseless against millions of organisms that can enter our bodies without detection, propagate and inflict damage to tissues.

As we all know, traditional modern medicine treats symptoms without going to the root of the condition. Most diseases are mainly caused by an immune system imbalance. By treating (for example) headaches, trouble sleeping, and muscle pain separately, we can successfully rid ourselves of the symptoms. However, this type of approach to an illness does not target the real problem, which could be stress, and, as we now know, stress is a very common illness, that depresses the immune system.

It is very important to use a holistic treatment for all diseases. Each organ does not function by itself without interacting with the rest of the organs. We are a complex system that needs to be viewed and treated as a whole.

One question that arises from all this is: How do I know when my immune system is not functioning properly? To find out if your immune system is up to par, you should look for the following signs of immune weakness: You catch a cold more then once a year, wounds or cuts take too long to heal, or they get infected frequently, you easily get fungal infections like Athlete's foot or candidiasis, you suffer from yeast infections, herpes, urinary tract infections or respiratory tract infections, fatigue, or lack of energy. These are all symptoms that can give you a hint that your immune system is in trouble or not in balance.

But the question is...How do we keep our immune system in balance and ready to tackle any disease?

Vitamin A, C, B, and E deficiencies have been linked to immune system weakness, so it is recommended that this vitamin be taken as part of a high potency multi-vitamin supplement. A proper diet, rich in vegetables, and low in chemicals or preservatives is essential to maintain the immune system at full strength. The excessive use of concentrated sugars (like syrups, honey), saturated fats, hormone and chemically treated foods have a detrimental effect on the immune system. Stress and lack of exercise can impair immune functioning.

A natural immune Booster.

Echinacea is a beautiful purple flower plant that grows in the United States and Europe. Its popularity goes beyond the reach of any other herb, not because of its beauty but because its properties. Echinacea is the herb of choice to treat any type of infectious disease. It's powerful and has no dangerous or harmful side effects. So far more then 400 studies have been done on Echinacea, each showing successful treatments of infectious diseases. Without a doubt it is one of my favorite herbs.

If you are serious at all in your desire to maintain and better your health, you must have some Echinacea in your medicine cabinet. There are literally millions of microbes, viruses, bacterium, and fungi; a simple cold can be caused by more then 200 different viruses. So, as you can imagine, our immune systems are very busy workers, and with such an immense amount of eager invaders, it is not surprising that many of these microorganisms make it through, and that's how we become ill with colds, flu, bronchitis, strep throat and many infectious diseases.

If you have read my book you know all the side effects caused by prescription and over the counter drugs used to treat these diseases. Nearly all these medications are toxic, and all of them are expensive.

Echinacea is a powerful, safe, and inexpensive remedy. But I believe its best attribute consists in the way it works with the immune system, bringing it to balance. It can be taken internally or applied externally on wounds and burns. It stimulates the activity of leukocytes, white blood cells that fight infection, and T lymphocytes or T cells; it increases the activity of macrophages, white cells that kill and eat harmful microorganisms, plus it has antibiotic properties and speeds up wound healing by encouraging healthy cell growth.

Echinacea has been popular for hundreds of years. It was named in the 1700's, but used by Native Americans for hundreds of years before that. Its popularity reached the European Continent and studies were done showing results that convinced even the most skeptical scientists. However, with the arrival of modern medicine to the U.S. and all its financial and political support, Echinacea and all the other herbs were regarded as old fashion and primitive. In Europe where doctors always believed that herbs are an important part of medicine Echinacea is still highly valued. European pharmacies carry a wide variety of herbal remedies. A rise in the popularity of Echinacea started again in the 1980's as people started to worry about the shortcomings of traditional medicine with regard to diseases like AIDS, Cancer, and many others that still have very high levels of mortality.

Today Echinacea and herbs in general are back in vogue. The use of herbal and home remedies is no longer regarded as outdated, and this means that in the future we might be able to enjoy a more affordable health system, as they do in Europe.

R.D.A's

This is a very important subject so let get started, shall we?

The numbers given by the Nutrition Board are a recommendation as to what Americans should be eating and how much in order to maintain their health. These recommendations are broken down into genders and age groups. For example, The RDA for a male fifty years of age is not the same as the RDA for a female 20 years of age.

RDAs are distinct from, but related to, the Reference Daily Intake (RDI) developed by the Food and Drug Administration to be used in food labelling. RDI replaced the term U.S. Recommended Daily Allowances which was used until new food labelling regulations went into effect in late 1992. All packaged foods were required to bear the new term on labels as of May 1994.
Because RDAs and RDIs are widely used, it is important to understand generally how to interpret them. The recommended allowances for nutrients are amounts intended to be consumed as part of a normal diet and are neither minimum requirements nor optimal levels of intake; it is not possible based on current research to set such specific guidelines nor to set a specific amount that would apply to all individuals. Rather, RDAs are safe and adequate levels of intake that reflect current knowledge.

Unfortunately most people don't eat well, not even the recommended amounts, this is the main cause of deficiency. Experts believe that many of the diseases affecting the average person are the result of not taking the necessary amount of nutrients needed to maintain a good health.

The problem is the complexity of the RDA table, for example, a child between 0 and 5 years of age needs 375 mg. of vitamin A, 7.5 mg. of vitamin D, 3 mg. of vitamin E, 5 mg. of vitamin K, 30 mg. of vitamin C, etc, etc, etc. and that's only for ages 0 - 5. As you can see there is no way to tell how much Vitamin D your child is taking a day or how much Iron is in the chicken your child had for lunch. The same problem is found in the RDA tables for men and women.

That is why I recommend the use of another method. The best way to know if you are getting the Recommended Dietary Allowance (RDA) for all the nutrients you need is to follow the Food guide pyramid. It provides from 1600 to over 2800 calories per day depending on which foods and the number of servings you eat. The assumption is made that if you will choose a variety of foods from each of the 5 food groups (Grain, Vegetable, Fruit, Milk, Meat) then you will probably get 100% of your RDA.

The Food Guide Pyramid is a tool used to teach people to eat a balanced diet from a variety of food portions without counting calories or any other nutrient. The USDA expanded the four food groups to six and expanded the number of servings to meet the calorie needs of most persons.

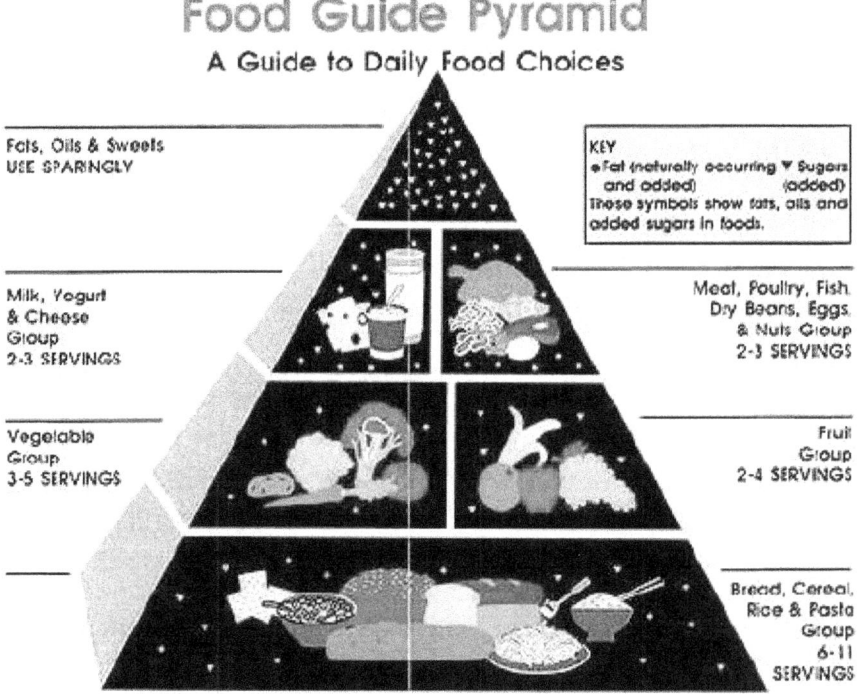

The Top of the Pyramid

Fats, oils and sweets should be used sparingly in the diet and therefore are represented as the small tip of the pyramid. This includes salad dressings, oils, cream, butter, margarine, soft drinks, candies and sweet desserts. These foods provide calories but little or no vitamins and minerals.

The Middle of the Pyramid

40

Protein is needed in moderate amounts in the diet and therefore represents the upper middle of the pyramid. Milk, yogurt, cheese, meat, poultry, fish, dry beans, eggs and nuts - two groups of foods that come mostly from animals - are important for protein, calcium, iron and zinc. Choose lean meats, skinless poultry, fish and low-fat dairy products to control fat and cholesterol. Also, limit breaded or fried foods to control fat and calories.

Most Americans need to eat more fruits and vegetables which helps form the foundation of the pyramid. Besides being an excellent source of vitamins, minerals and fiber, vegetables and fruits (plant foods) are low-fat, low-sodium and cholesterol-free.
Eating a variety of vegetables and fruits will help ensure that you meet your daily need for Vitamin C and other nutrients.

The Base of the Pyramid

Bread, cereals, rice and pasta - all foods from grains - are found at the base of the Pyramid because they are the foundation upon which the rest of the diet is planned. Try to choose 6-11 servings daily. Grains supply fiber, carbohydrates, vitamins and minerals. They are usually low in fat and are the preferred fuel for our brain, nervous system and muscles. To keep these foods low in fat and calories, limit the use of spreads.

The information in this brochure was adapted from USDA's Food Guide Pyramid, US Department of Agriculture, Human Nutrition Information Service, 1992.

What Counts as One Serving?

Here are some serving size examples for each food group. If you eat a larger portion, count it as more than one serving.

Most Americans are encouraged to eat at least the lowest number of servings from the five food groups each day.

Bread, Cereal, Rice and Pasta Group (6-11 servings)

   1 slide of bread

  · 1 ounce of ready-to-eat cereal (check labels: 1 ounce = 1/4 cup to 2 cups depending on cereal)

  · 1/2 cup of cooked cereal, rice or pasta

  · 1/2 hamburger roll, bagel, English muffin

· 3 or 4 plain crackers (small)

Vegetable Group (3-5 servings)

· 1 cup of raw leafy vegetables

· 1/2 cup of other vegetables, cooked or chopped raw

· 3/4 cup of vegetable juice

Fruit Group (2-4)

· 1 medium apple, banana, orange, nectarine, peach

· 1/2 cup of chopped, cooked or canned fruit

· 3/4 cup of fruit juice

Milk, Yogurt, and Cheese Group (2-3 servings)

· 1 cup of milk or yogurt

· 1.5 ounces of natural cheese

· 2 ounces of processed cheese

Meat, Poultry, Fish, Dry Beans, Eggs, and Nuts Group (2-3 servings)

· 2 to 3 ounces of cooked lean meat, poultry or fish

· (1 ounce of meat = 1/2 cup of cooked dry beans, 1 egg or 2 tablespoons of peanut butter)

How Much Should I Eat?

1200 calories is the lowest amount recommended to maintain nutritional adequacy; this calorie level is conducive for weight loss or extremely inactive individuals.

1600 calories is recommended for many sedentary women and some older adults.

2200 calories is recommended for most children, teenage girls, active women and sedentary men; women who are pregnant or breast feeding may need more.

2500 calories is recommended for teenage boys, active men and some very active women.

Injuries

We are always careful that our kids don't hurt themselves or fearful that something might happen to one of us. That's why we have a complete first aid kit but is there anything in that kit to help with burns or poisoning chances are there isn't.

So that's when a home remedy comes handy. In this section we will help you treat many of the common household injuries that can ruin your day.

Anything from a bruise to a broken bone, a cut or bee sting, can be treated with natural healing products. Sure you will need to go to a hospital for many of these injuries but using natural remedies before and after the visit to the doctor, can improve the recovery process and help speed up healing.

Chances are you have a first aid kit in your home. I recommend you add the following herbals to your kit; this way you´ll always have an herbal alternative to treat injuries and conditions. The herbs suggested for first-aid are safe and effective and generally cause few of the side effects normally associated with pharmaceutical drugs. As with any medicine, though, you should keep these remedies out of the reach of young children who often eat anything that comes within their reach.

The Herbal First Aid Kit

Aloe
Break off an aloe leaf and scrape the gel to soothe minor burns, scalds, and sunburns. Aloe has tissue regenerative properties and will help heal all wounds.

Arnica
Arnica cream or oil can be used on bruises or sprains where the skin is not broken. Caution should be used with Arnica however since it can become toxic in high doses.

Calendula Cream
Homemade or storebought, this is antispetic and antifungal. If you

make it, try adding comfrey to the cream; it will help speed the healing process.

Clove Oil
Clove oil is an excellent antispetic for cuts and is also useful for treating toothaches. It should be cut with a carrier oil when used on the skin since severe irritation can occur.

Compresses
Keep squares of gauze or cheesecloth on hand to make compresses. Use comfrey, witch hazel, or arnica for sprains; St. John's Wort for deep cuts; comfrey or witch hazel for burns.

Crystallized Ginger
Chew for motion sickness or morning sickness.

Eucalyptus Oil
This is a good inhalant for colds, coughs, and respiratory infections.

Rescue Remedy
This combination of 5 of the Bach Flower Remedies is effective for shocks and emotional upsets, especially in children.

St. John's Wort Infused Oil
Excellent for minor burns and sunburn.

Slippery Elm
Slippery elm powder is used to make poultices for drawing out splinters and bringing boils to a head.

Tea Tree Oil
Antispetic and antifungal. Useful for cleansing wounds.

Witch Hazel Extract
Use it to treat minor burns, sunburn, and insect bites. Apply to nasal passages to stop nosebleeds. Wash cuts with it to help cleanse them.

Please remember to follow up on any serious injuries with a qualified physician.

> TIP: A home made ice pack can be made by mixing 2 parts water and 1 part alcohol in a nylon bag and freezing it. The bag will be flexible thus molding to the body and it will not sweat.

Bee Sting and insect bite:

Everything from a mosquito to a spider can cause serious reactions in the body. The problem is not the injury but what the insect leaves behind (the venom). This is a defense mechanism that is used when, for example, a beehive detects danger.

When someone is stung by an insect, the area becomes swollen, red, extremely painful or burning. However some people may be allergic to some insects, which can cause even more dangerous symptoms like hard to breathe, hard to swallow, disorientation, swelling of eyes and mouth or unconsciousness. These cases must be treated urgently by a professional.

Nature gives us hundreds of insects that can bite or sting, but it also gives us an array of herbs that can reduce the itching and swelling, we are even going to show you how to make your own natural repellent as well. While we do not have any studies to show if herbal repellents are better than their commercial counter parts, they certainly smell better and we don't think you would want to rub toxic chemicals on your body.

The earth is in balance, mother nature produces everything we need, it is up to us to prepare and use what is given.

We recommend:

* Remove the stinger. Do Not squeeze it, this will inject more of the venom in the patient.

* Clean the area.

* Crush Plantain leaves extracting the juice and applying it on the injured area.

* Apply toothpaste on the sting.

* A homeopathic remedy that can be very helpful is Apis Mallifica, 30x. It reduces inflammation and pain, burning and stinging.

TIP: Did you know that granulated sugar can be used to prevent scarring of a bite wound?

* A homeopathic remedy called Cantharis 30c is good for bee or wasp stings.

* A homeopathic remedy called Carbolicum acidum 30c is used in more severe allergic reactions to bee stings or black widow spider bites.

* A homeopathic remedy called Urtica urens 30c is good for itching, burning and pain.

Insect bite lotion.

1 teaspoon lavender essential oil
1 tablespoon vegetable oil
Combine essential oil and vegetable oil and dab mixture directly on bite as needed. Store in a bottle with a tight lid. A glass container is best, but if you prefer a lighter, plastic container, choose one made of oil-resistant plastic (you can find these in camping goods stores). Make sure to keep the Insect Bite Oil away from your eyes.

* Lavender stops itching and reduces swelling.

Extra strength sting poultice.

1 tbs.. echinacea root tincture.
1 tbs.. distilled water.
1/8 tsp. lavender essential oil.
1 tbs.. bentonite clay.
Mix the echinacea, water and lavender. Add liquid slowly to the clay while stirring. Once mixed, the resulting paste should stick to the skin. Apply on the injured area. Store the poultice in a tight lid container, if it does dry out, add water until moist enough to stick to

the skin.

TIP: Did you know that a slice of raw onion placed on an animal bite will discourage infection   and draw poison out?

* Jewelweed is used to reduce itching and soothe the skin, take two or three leaves, break them and apply the juice over the injured area.

Ant and nettle medicine.

The allergic reaction from a bite or a sting is caused by formic acid which can be neutralized using 1 tsp. of yellow dock leaf tincture and 2 tsp. of baking soda. Mix the ingredients and form a poultice. Apply as needed.

Home made Insect repellents.

2 ounces of vodka.
1/4 tsp. citronella essential oil.
1/4 tsp. eucalyptus essential oil.
1/8 tsp. pennyroyal essential oil. (Do not use during pregnancy)
1/8 tsp. cedar essential oil.
1/8 tsp. rose geranium essential oil.
Mix the ingredients and apply it on the exposed skin. Keep away from the mouth and eyes.

Insect Repellent 2

2 ounces vodka
¼ teaspoon each citronella and eucalyptus essential oils
1/8 teaspoon each pennyroyal, cedar and rose geranium essential oils
Combine ingredients and apply mixture directly to all exposed skin. Keep away from eyes and mouth.

Note: Conventional repellents are toxic chemicals. Homemade herbal repellents have a more pleasant fragrance than the ones sold in drugstore, therefore using them is certainly preferable.

Topical wash for bites and stings.

2 tsp. confrey leaves.
2 tbs.. marshmallow leaves.
1 tbs.. dried yarrow.
1 cup of boiling water.
Mix herbs and cover with boiling water. Steep for 30 minutes, strain.
Wash area with this solution 4 times a day.

Fast healing ointment.

1 pound petroleum jelly.
4 tbs.. of agrimony leaves.
4 tsp. dried marigold flowers.
Melt jelly using steam, add the herbs and heat for 1 hour, strain.
Apply as needed.

Other natural insect repellents.

Use any of the following tinctures.

For bees Apis mellifica, Ledum, or Urnica urens.
For gnat Calendula or Hypericum.
For wasp Arnica or Ledum.
For mosquitos Staphysagria 12c can be taken orally.

Mice Repellent.

Here's a quick tip for making sachets that will actually keep mice out.

Take some old pantyhose and fill them with dried, crushed peppermint leaves. Tie up the bags securely and toss a few under the beds, in closets and even in the stove and dishwasher.

Squirrels can become unwelcome guests, too, but if you find them in your attic or chimney, just reach for the aftershave. It may smell great to you, but it's repulsive to squirrels. They'll be saying good bye in no time.

Bone Fracture:

When a bone in the body breaks or cracks it's called a fracture. There are two types of fractures: closed or open. When the skin that covers the bone remains intact that is a closed fracture. When the bone breaks the skin, that is a open or compound fracture.
When a fracture occurs, it causes terrible pain and tenderness in the area fractured, along with swelling, the appearance of some blood under the skin and some numbness, tingling or paralysis below the injured area.

When a person fractures an arm or leg, he or she could lose the pulse below the fracture. Fractures are more common in young children and in older adults. As we grow older, our bones get weaker and more fragile, and they take more and more time to heal themselves.

A fracture requires professional attention, what we offer here are recommendations that will aid in healing after the bone has been set.

We recommend

*Eat half a pineapple every day until the fracture completely healed. Pineapple contains Bromelain, an enzyme that helps reduce swelling and inflammation. Do not eat canned or processed pineapples. If you don't like fresh pineapple, take the supplement Bromelain. It has the same effect as pineapple.

*Do not eat red meat, and avoid drinking colas and all products containing caffeine.

*Avoid eating foods with preservatives, they contain Phosphorous which can lead to bone loss.

*Take Boron, it is important for the health and healing of the bone.

*Take Calcium + Magnesium + Potassium. They are essential to repair bone damage and to maintain a good muscle and heart condition.

*Take Zinc, it helps repair tissue damage.

*Vitamin C with bioflavonoids. It is very important for the restoration of bones, connective tissue and muscles.

*Vitamin D3 helps to prevent fractures, and is needed for the absorption of calcium.

*Octacosonal improves tissue connection.

*Vitamin B complex + Vitamin B5, help maintain healthy muscle tone and proper brain function. For an older adult it is very important to take these vitamins because these nutrients are very difficult to absorb as we age.

*Horsetail extract contains silica which enhances the utilization of calcium and promotes healing and repair.

*The herb Broswellia helps one to recover faster after a fracture, easing pain and acting as an anti-inflammatory. It's as effective as ibuprofen.

*Use Comfrey in fractures. It reduces pain and cuts bone healing time in half. It can be used in amputation. It's excellent for bone bruising and skull injuries.

*Eat lots of carrots. They are rich in vitamin A needed to make the broken area stronger.

Bruising:

A bruise or contusion is an injury to the tissue under the skin caused by a blow from an object. The skin does not break but the blood vessels that run throughout out our bodies rupture, and blood drains into the tissue, seeping into the skin. This causes pain, swelling, and a characteristic discoloration of the skin (black and blue colors). Some people become bruised very easily, sometimes even without evidence of trauma, this is caused by lack of vitamin C, and nutrients found in fresh foods (vegetable and fruits), without theses vitamins and minerals, blood vessels become weak and thin, prone to rupture when light pressure is applied. Other reason could be diabetes, or menstruation. If the bruise does not go away check with your doctor, it might be a sign of a more serious condition.

Some modern medicines, such as antidepressants, aspirin, anesthetics, cortisone and penicillin, can interfere with normal blood clotting, thus causing bruises to appear.

We recommend

TIP: A home made ice pack can be made by mixing 2 parts water and 1 part alcohol in a nylon bag and freezing   it. The bag will be flexible thus molding to the body and it will not sweat.

*Take Vitamin K or alfalfa in tablets helps blood clotting.

*Take Vitamin C to prevent bruising by thickening the walls of blood vessels.

*Make a tea with confrey root or buchu soak a rag in the tea and apply to bruised area. This has been shown to reduce pain and discoloration of the skin.

*Fresh parsley crushed is very helpful when placed on injured area.

*Place an ice pack immediately after injury has occur, keep it in place for 20 minutes. This contracts the blood vessels thus stopping the internal bleeding.

*Eat lots of fruits, chicken and eggs (rich in zinc), broccoli, cabbage, spinach (rich in vitamin K).

*Do not take Aspirin or ibuprofen (Advil etc.) for pain. These medicines contain blood thinners that can make the bruise bigger and darker. You could take Tylenol instead.

*Take the homeopathic remedy Arnica in tablets. In Germany pharmacies carry more then 100 different kinds of arnica preparations for different kinds of injuries.

TIP : If the bruise is under a fingernail or a toe take Hypericum. This is a good remedy for bruises on extremities and areas of the body rich in nerve endings.

*Saint John's Wort tincture is great to remove bruises in one or two days.

Bruise compress.

1 tbs. of arnica flowers tincture.
1 tbs. of Saint John's Wort tincture.
1 tbs. of witch hazel bark tincture.
1 tbs. of chamomile flowers tincture.
4 drops of lavender essential oil.
2 tbs. of cold water.
1 cotton cloth.
Combine the ingredients and soak the cloth in it. Wring it out and apply on the bruises. To make an extra cold and extra strength compress add the herbal ice listed below.

Herbal ice.

1 cup of water.
1 tsp. of chamomile flowers.

1 tsp. lavender flowers.
Pour boiling water on herbs and let it steep for 30 minutes, strain and place in an ice tray, freeze. Place inside the bruise compress.

*Mustard or black pepper oil draws blood away from the bruise.

*Roasted onion in a poultice helps bruising.

*Chinese people use a mixture of 1 part cayenne pepper and 5 parts melted Vaseline, mix and cool, apply once a day.

Burns:

A burn is a very traumatic injury caused by fire, chemicals, steam, electricity or any other form of heat transfer to the skin (our biggest organ). Burns on less then 10% of the body surface are considered minor. An entire hand is 1% of the body surface. There are three types of burns and they are classified by their severity. First degree burns are the ones to the top layers of the skin. The area becomes red and painful. Sunburn is an example of a first degree burn. Second degree burns are the ones that go deeper damaging more layers of skin. The skin becomes red and extremely painful with blisters. Third degree burns are the most serious of them all. The entire thickness of the skin is destroyed and in some cases muscle and other tissues are damaged. There is little pain involved as most of the nerves are burned and the brain is unable to sense pain. The skin turns red or white and without proper care the area may become infected sometimes turning yellow or black. In severe burns a skin graft may be needed.

*IMPORTANT*Do not attempt to treat a third degree burn yourself. These types of injury are life threatening and they require professional attention. Natural remedies can help after hospitalization to prevent infection and boost immune system defenses.

In minor burns herbs and homeopathic medicines have remarkable success reliving pain and speeding up healing.

We recommend

Use some of these techniques to treat burns:

*Apply Colloidal silver. It is a natural antibiotic and disinfectant. If the burn is very painful, use in spray.

*Apply a lotion made with vitamin A.

*Take Vitamin C w/ bioflavonoids which is an antioxidant needed for the formation of collagen. Studies have shown that high doses of vitamin C are very necessary.

*Take vitamin E as needed to prevent scarring.

*Aloe vera applied directly to the burned area to relieve pain and speed healing.

*Calendula lotion and cantharis in tablets are very good homeopathic remedies for burns.

A poultice is very helpful prepared as follows:
1 tablespoon of dried coneflower flowers.
1 tablespoon of hyssop flowers.
1 tablespoon of goldenrod flowers.
1 tablespoon of dried sunflower petals.
Mix ingredients and soak them with boiling water, let cool, place between gauze and apply on burned area, re moistening as needed.

*Apply fresh ginger juice to burn with cotton.

*Goldenseal in form of extract should be used externally. It's a natural antibiotic and prevents infections.

*Horsetail helps skin heal faster.

*Immerse the burned area in cold water with a few drops of Hypericum or Urtica urens. Never use butter or Vaseline, ice water or ice cubes on a burn.

TIP: Do not puncture blisters caused by burns. They provide a barrier against bacteria that can cause infection.

*If clothing is stuck to the skin do not remove it.

*Look for infection in the days after a burn, if pus or a bad odor is detected use remedies recommended.

*For acid or chemical burns use baking soda or apple cider vinegar added to warm water.

*Crush blueberries and extract the juice. Apply using cotton balls.

*Raw potatoes cut in slices and applied directly on the burn provide instant relief.

*A few drops of echinacea tincture in a liter of water, and poured over the burn helps prevent infection.

*Add Marigold tincture to the gauze that covers the burn. This will speed up healing.

*Lavender is great to kill germs and improve healing time.

*Boil a liter of water, let it cool and add a few drops of geranium oil. Pour over the burn to encourage healing.

Treatment for blisters.

*Apply aloe vera juice to the blisters to improve healing.

*If the blister is infected, apply barberry.

*Bathe the blister with salty water. This will discourage the growth of bacteria thus preventing infection.

*For infected blisters, a poultice of roasted onions has been shown to improve the condition.

*Witch hazel applied to blisters will reduce pain, swelling and speed up healing.

*If blisters break, clean the surrounding area and the open blisters with a few drops of Roman chamomile and water.

Dog Bite:

When an animal scratches or bites braking the skin, a number of problems can arise, the most important is infection caused by the animal's saliva. A dog bite may be a minor injury or a severe attack especially in children.
If a dog bites, you should immediately demand from the dog´s owner proof of immunization. Rabies is very dangerous and it can kill if not treated in time. If the dog is foaming from the mouth that is a sign of rabies. If you don't know the owner of the dog, the animal should be caught in order to be tested for diseases.

There is also risk of tetanus in all puncture injuries. Never run from a dog it stimulates the animal's instincts to chase and bite.

We recommend:

* Wash the dog bite thoroughly with warm water and soap for more then 5 minutes to remove the saliva. Rinse with cold water and place a gauze on the wound.

* Take Vitamin C. It helps fight infection.

* Take vitamin B. It helps to produce antibodies.

* If the bite is big, see a doctor, it might be necessary for the wound to be stitched.

* Take Echinacea in tea form.

* Drinking Goldenseal tea on the first day of the injury is very good for dog bites. Do not use this if you are pregnant.

* Goldenseal applied directly on the bite is helpful as a natural antibiotic.

Here's a quick tip for making sachets that will actually keep mice out.

Take some old pantyhose and fill them with dried, crushed peppermint leaves. Tie up the bags securely and toss a few under the beds, in closets and even in the stove and dishwasher.

Squirrels can become unwelcome guests, too, but if you find them in your attic or chimney, just reach for the aftershave. It may smell great to you, but it's repulsive to squirrels. They'll be saying good-bye in no time.

Poison Ivy, Oak and Sumac:

These three plants are responsible for more cases of dermatitis than any other substances. When contact is made with any part of the plant a rash develops on the skin. This rash is caused by a reaction to a chemical compound in the resin called urushiol (one of the most potent toxins on earth) found all over the plant. Some cases have been reported from people who came in contact with pets that had been in the bushes. When the plant is burned, the smoke is also an irritant and can cause a reaction in the respiratory tract.

The symptoms are red pimples that are extremely itchy, swelling, blisters, burning, inflammation, fever and/or inflamation in the face or genital area. The appearance of the symptoms can be between anywhere from a few hours to seven or ten days after contact with the plant. It can then spread rapidly during the next three days, especially with scratching.

The areas most likely to be affected by poison ivy are the hands, arms, face or legs. Scratching the rash can spread the inflammation to other parts of the body. Redness, swelling and itching usually begin to heal after the second day that the rash appears.

Normally a person can be completely healed within seven to fourteen days of coming into contact with poison ivy.

Direct contact with the plant is the most common way to contract poison ivy but it can also be contracted if a person pets an animal or touches a cloth or object that has been in contact with the plant in some way. Some people who are extremely sensitive to poison ivy can develop a reaction if the plant is burned and they inhale the smoke. Children who have eaten the plant's leaves or their grayish berries had severe mouth poisoning.

We recommend:

* Take Vitamin C with bioflavonoids to help to prevent infection and the rapid spreading of the rash caused by poison ivy and reduces swelling.

* Take Calcium and Beta-carotene as they help to boost the immune response and speed healing of poison ivy.

* Take Zinc. It helps repair skin tissue damaged by poison ivy.

* Use Calamine lotion. It is good for speed healing of poison ivy.

* Use Vitamin E oil or cream. It is effective to prevent scars and help healing.

* Take Vitamin A with mixed caroteriods to help repair skin tissue and boost the immune system.

* Eat a diet rich in sea vegetables to provide the body with tons of immune-boosting minerals.

* Avoid consuming sugar, fried foods and fats.

* To treat any case of poison ivy, try one or more of the following treatments:

Apply cool water compresses mixed with one tsp. of sea salt per pint of water over blisters and crusts to calm. Leave the compresses for 15 minutes, repeating the procedure for a few hours until itching is gone.

Taking cool oatmeal, salt or diluted vinegar baths also reduce itching. After the bath, dry the affected area with a blow dryer. That will reduce the itching even more.

Another way to reduce itching is mixing one tsp. of water with 3 tsp. of one of these dry ingredients; cornstarch, baking soda, oatmeal or Epson salts. Make a paste and apply over the affected skin.

For cooling relief, apply over the itching area aloe vera juice, tofu or watermelon rind. They soothe and dry poison ivy immediately.

Calendula lotion is very good in reducing itching, limiting the spread of the rash and helping the body heal faster.

Mix any or all of these ingredients and make a tea to detoxify the body: burdock, nettle, red clover and yellow dock. Drink a cup of tea 3 or 4 times a day until rash is gone.

Try any of these essential oils to soothe inflamed skin, reduce itching and to relieve anxiety: benzoin, cedarwood,chamomile, everlasting, geranium, jasmine, juniper, lavender, neroli, orange, patchouli, peppermint, rose, rosemary,
rosewood, sandalwood, tea tree, thyme, and ylang ylang. Use them in baths, compresses and body oil.

Here are some homeopathic remedies for poison ivy:

If your face is affected by the rash, take Anacardium.

If you only have blisters in the palm of your hands, take Anagallis.

If the face is involved and the eyelids are swollen, take Apis mellifica.

If the genital area or the scalp is affected, take Croton tiglium.

If you have any asthmatic symptoms and your skin is purplish and swollen, take Grindelia.

If the itching has a burning sensation, take Sulfur.

Sunburn:

Sunburn is caused by excessive exposure to the sun's ultraviolet (UV) rays. The sun's ultraviolet rays are the ones responsible when we have a sunburn. There are two types of ultraviolet rays: ultraviolet A (UVA) and ultraviolet B (UVB). Both are very strong and harmful to the skin. UVB rays attack the skin's outer layers while UVA are rays that attack the underlying layers.

When they are reflected on water, metal, snow, or sand their effects intensifies. The intensity of a sunburn depends of the amount of exposure from the individual, the geographical location, the time, and the atmospheric conditions. Sunburns, like any other burn, are classified as first degree, second degree and third degree. Normally, sunburns are first degree burns.

The symptoms of a first degree burn include pain, heat, redness and tenderness to the touch in the skin affected. These symptoms can appear from 1 to 24 hours after exposure to the sun. After a couple of days this type of burn will "cool" into a suntan or thin layers of skin may peel off.

The symptoms of a second degree burn include extreme reddening, swelling, pain and even blisters can appear. The burn goes deeper into the skin's layers damaging small blood vessels and elastic fibers in the skin and later there is wrinkling of the skin. In most severe cases, the burn may be accompanied by chills, fever, nausea, and/or delirium. Sunburn such as this is extremely painful and for children it's terribly dangerous.

Today, the effects of sun exposure is a common concern because of the decline in the earth's ozone layer. The ozone's layers are what protects us from harmful UV rays which damages our skin and causes many diseases like skin cancer.

We recommend:

* Take measures to prevent yourself from getting sunburned:

* Avoid being outdoors between 10:00 am and 3:00 pm, when the UV rays are more intense.

* If you have to be outside during these hours, try to wear a hat, sunglasses that protect your eyes from UV rays and clothing made of light colored, light weight, tightly woven material.

* Use a sunscreen with a sun protection factor (SPF) of 15 or higher. Apply to the skin whenever you go outside or ride in the car. Apply it to all exposed areas 30 minutes before going outside, repeating the procedure as often as possible, especially if you are swimming or perspiring. Make sure you buy a sunscreen that contains protection against both UVA and UVB rays.

* Take the same precautions on cloudy or foggy days as you do on bright, sunny days. Approximately 80% of the sun's UV rays pass through the clouds.

* Always protect your lips, they are very susceptible to sunburn. Using a sun protection product designed for the lips and made of natural ingredients such as aloe vera and vitamin E.

* To prevent free radical damage to the skin, add to your sunscreen 1 capsule of Vitamin A, Vitamin C, Vitamin E, and Selenium. You can also add these Vitamins to your moisturizer for extra protection and to prevent wrinkles.

* Drink plenty of fluids to prevent dehydration.

* Eat lots of lean and high quality protein foods. Also include raw fruits to supply the vitamins and minerals needed.

* Eat plenty of green and yellow vegetables. They contain Vitamin C and Beta carotene and they help build new connective tissue and strengthen the blood vessels.

* Eat pumpkin seeds and oysters. They are a good source of zinc.

* Drink plenty of fluids to keep your body hydrated and to replace what is lost by the sunburn.

* To relieve sunburn pain, apply over the affected area cool water compresses or fill a bathtub with cold water and dissolve a pound of baking soda or oatmeal in it. Soak in the bath for 30 minutes approximately or until you feel relief.

* Wash the affected area with an antibacterial soap to prevent secondary infection.

* Do not burst any blister. They form a natural protection to help the sunburned skin heal faster.

* Do not apply any creams, butter, petroleum jelly or any other greasy substance to a sunburn. They only cause more damage by trapping the heat and can make a burn deeper. The sunburn will heal faster if left exposed to the air.

* Take Coenzyme Q10. It increases the supply of oxygen to the cells.

* Use Colloidal Silver. It prevents infection, reduces inflammation and promotes healing.

* Take L-Cysteine to accelerate the healing of burns.

* Take a multivitamin and mineral complex to supply the vitamins and minerals we do not receive through our food.

* Take Potassium to replace the potassium lost through sunburn.

* Take Vitamin A + carteriods to help repair the skin's tissue damaged by sunburn and to destroy free radicals released by sun exposure.

* Take Vitamin C + bioflavonoids. They repair the skin's damaged tissue and reduce scaring.

* Take zinc to boosts the immune system and help heal damage skin.

* Apply Aloe Vera on the damaged skin, several times a day until the pain is gone. If you can, try to apply the gel directly from fresh plant to ease the discomfort caused by sunburn and to keep the burn from turning white and blistering. The Aloe Vera gel decreases pain, reduces inflammation, speeds wound healing, and has antibacterial and antifungal properties. It increases the amount of blood to the sunburned area, speeding healing and stimulating new skin cell growth. If you buy a commercial Aloe product, make sure that it contains no mineral oil, paraffin waxes, alcohol, or coloring.

* Apply Calendula cream directly to the sunburn to relieve discomfort, inflammation and pain. It also has antiseptic properties and prevents scaring.

* Apply St. Jonh's Wort tincture directly to the sunburn. It has the same properties as Calendula cream. Or you can make an oil by mixing 1 or 2 tsp. of the dried herb with a few ounces of vegetable oil and apply to the sunburn until you feel relief.

* Fill a bathtub with lukewarm water and add 6 cups of Chamomile tea or 6 drops of Chamomile oil (you can use Lavender instead of Chamomile if desired). Soak for 30 minutes or more to minimize the pain of sunburn.

* Make a tea using the herb Comfrey. Do not drink it, soak cotton in it and apply to the sunburn.

* Taking silica in capsules is very necessary to repair tissue.

* Rub Tea tree oil in lotion form on the sunburn.

Home remedies for Children

As parents, when our children get sick one of the first things we want to do is to run to the doctor. Other people start dosing their children with everything in the medicine cabinet. Needless to say neither of the two alternatives is the correct one. Even physicians agree lately that prescribing antibiotics and other drugs is not recommended for children. However, doctors sometime feel pressure by the parents to prescribe something even though he or she knows that the condition will disappear in a few days without drug intervention.

In most children a middle ear infection clears up on its own within a few months yet 90% of doctors will prescribe an antibiotic for this condition just to make the parent feel that the visit was time and money well spent.

Most ailments that affect children can be treated with over the counter medicine but many professionals are questioning the long term effects of giving synthetic drugs to a child from a very early age. Besides if the condition is treatable with over the counter drugs, no doubt herbs can do a better job and by using herbs you get peace of mind knowing that the problem is being taken care of and that you are boosting your child´s immune system without side effects. In my case, I feel very proud of myself every time my son gets better thanks to some herb preparation I made for him and it makes me happy to know that I choose to keep my child chemical free as much as I can.

But lets face it, children will run away every time they need to take a medicine made of herbs and soon you find yourself running around the table trying to catch the patient. There is a better way. herb preparation can be made in a way that children look forward to. By following the steps and instructions in this part of the book you will learn how to make a sweet tasting cough syrup, a spray for sore throats, a delicious tea for indigestion and if your baby is allergic to rash prevention products, we'll show you how to make your own totally natural baby powder, diaper rash cream, and baby oil. For more serious ailments you'll learn how to make your own infection fighting antibiotic by mixing the right herbs. Also you'll find formulas to make laxatives for your child's constipation and also how to make ear drops.

DOSAGE

Kids come in all sizes so it is very hard to know how much medicine is enough and how much is too much. So we will use a table that gives you the exact the amount of medicine you need to give to your child according to your child's weight.
Although throughout the book we recommend a dose for each remedy, this is for children whose weight is between 36 and 65 pounds. For kids that are either lighter or heavier, follow the instructions below.

WEIGHT	DOSAGE
Up to 5 pounds	1/16 cup/1tbsp.
5 to 15 pounds	1/8 cup / 2tbsp.
16 to 35 pounds	1/4 cup / 4tbsp.
36 to 65 pounds	½ cup
66 to 80 pounds	3/4 cup
81 to 110 pounds	1 cup

Most books show you what herbs can do. Some talk about herbs without going deeply into the subject of disease treating and I'm yet to find a book that offers true herbal remedies for children. If anyone should benefit from the properties of herbs it is your child. Scientists and doctors are becoming very concerned that our children are being over medicated, partly because the anxiety of the parent who expects to walk out of the doctor's office with a prescription to treat the child.

The main problem with this method of treating childhood conditions is that later in life the viruses and bacteria could develop resistance to the drugs and antibiotics used indiscriminately early in life. Which means that more powerful drugs need to be used to treat the illness every time.

We all know that chemicals need to be removed from our lives as much as possible and children are the most affected by this type of chemical warfare that we have unleashed on ourselves. Our children are becoming more and more sensitive to chemicals because of exposure to pollutants and synthetics substances that can change the immune system and destroy defenses. Asthma, food allergies, skin conditions and other problems are on the rise probably due to the increased exposure to all these harmful chemicals and the chemicals passed down from the mother while pregnant.

There are many childhood diseases that can be treated with herbs and there are herbs that prevent disease and boost the immune system. If your child is often coming down with something the cure lies with the natural antibiotics and immune busters that can be grown in your own back yard.

Asthma (See also Asthma in Common illnesses)

Modern medicine can offer very little to children with asthma. Most drugs can only produce a temporary effect. Herbs on the other hand can be very helpful not only reducing attacks but also in strengthening the lungs and immune system. You'll learn to treat this disease with many combinations of herbs such as mullein, elecampane and more.

Improve Breathing.

1 quart boiling water.
1 tsp. chamomile flowers.
1 tsp. echinacea root.
1 tsp. mullein leaves.
1 tsp. passionflower leaves.
Mix all ingredients and steep for 15 minutes, strain and drink 1 cup a day.

A very tasteful herb for children is Lemon verbena tea. This herb reduces wheezing and doctors recommend it in South America.

Chinese Asthma Remedy.

1 tsp. magnolia flowers.
1 tsp. rehmannia root.
½ tsp. don quai root.
3 cups of water.
Mix ingredients steep for 10 minutes and strain. Drink 2 cups a day.

Home Made Chest Rub.

8 drops lavender essential oil.

2 drops chamomile essential oil.

1/4 cup of olive oil.

Mix ingredients. Rub on the chest as needed, ideally before bedtime.

Herbal Bronchial Steam.

2 cups of water.

3 drops of lavender essential oil.

2 drops chamomile essential oil.

Boil water, turn off heat and add essential oils. Place a towel over your head and over the pot, close your eyes and let the steam warm your face. Then after 15 minutes splash your face with cool water.

Diaper Rash Treatment.

Home Made Baby Powder.

½ pound cornstarch.

1/4 tsp. lavender essential oil.

Place the cornstarch in a self-sealing plastic bag and add the essential oil, mix and shake well breaking the lumps as they form. This will ensure that the oil is evenly spread. Store the bag in a warm dark and dry place for four days. If you don't want to use cornstarch, potato starch or arrowroot powder can be used as well.

Diaper Rash Cream.

1/4 cup of olive or vegetable oil.

5 drops calendula essential oil.

5 drops of elder essential oil.

½ ounce beeswax.

5 400 IU Vitamin E capsules.

2 1,000 IU Vitamin A capsules.

Mix oil with essential oils and wax, heat enough to melt the wax, puncture the capsules and squeeze the content into the oil and stir for a minute. Remove from heat and while the mixture is hot pour into a wide-mouthed container. Use on every diaper change.

Baby Oil.

½ cup dried lavender flowers.
½ cup dried calendula flowers.
½ cup dried elder flowers.
3 cups almond oil (or vegetable oil).
Chop all dried herbs and place them in a glass jar, cover herbs with oil and stir. Place a tight lid on the jar and place on top of a radiator or in a warm sunny place for three days. Strain the herbs using a coffee filter. Use as needed to treat rashes and as a massage oil.

Cradle Cap Remedy.

Cradle cap is a crusty rash that forms on the scalp and face of newborn babies. The only conventional treatment available uses cortisone. If you are like me, you would rather not use such a powerful steroid on a baby especially when herbs offer a much better alternative.

1/4 cup aloe vera.
3 drops lavender essential oil.
3 drops tea tree essential oil.
Mix ingredients in a plastic bottle shake very well. Apply on the head twice a day.

Immune System Booster.

If your child is suffering from a cold or flu or if you want to prevent him from getting any illness, your best option is to boost his or her immune system. This next remedy will keep your child healthy throughout winter. Also, it speeds up the recovery from mumps, chickenpox, flu and colds.

In a small town called Chirchik, Russia, a flu epidemic swept the town. When many adults and children did not get sick scientists wanted to know why they were immune to the disease. It turns out that all of them used the berries from an herb called Shizandra.

2 cups of water.
1 tsp. echinacea root.
½ tsp. chamomile leaves.
½ tsp. shizandra berries.
½ tsp. peppermint leaves.

Mix herbs pour boiling water over and steep for 10 minutes. Strain and drink 1 cup a day.

If these herbs are hard to find, you can make or buy the tinctures, use three drops of each.

Diarrhea.   (See also Diarrhea in Common Illnesses)

Children develop diarrhea frequently and the causes sometimes are different from those of adults. A child could suffer a bout of diarrhea simply by eating too fast, too much, or by eating foods that are too difficult for the young to digest. Also, intestinal flu and intolerance to some intestinal bacteria can cause diarrhea in children.

For adults it´s ok to use blackberry root but for children this can be too potent. Instead, the berries or leaves of the plant can be used to stop diarrhea in children but make sure to remove the seeds because they can act as a laxative which is the opposite result.

Children diarrhea tea.

3 cups of water.
1 tsp. catnip leaves.
½ tsp. raspberry or blackberry leaves.
½ tsp. slippery elm bark.
½ tsp. peppermint leaves.
½ tsp. cinnamon bark powder.
Mix ingredients and simmer for 5 minutes, remove from heat and steep for 20 minutes, strain and give several times a day.

Blackberry shake.

½ cup blackberry juice.
1 banana.
½ tsp. cinnamon bark powder.
1 tsp. sugar.
Blend in all ingredients, and serve. Your child will love it.

Rice preparation for diarrhea.

½ cup of rice.
2 cups of water.
1/4 tsp. Oregon grape root powdered.
½ tsp. cinnamon powder.
1 banana.
Boil rice and water until soft, (30 minutes). Blend rice, Oregon root powder and banana. Serve and sprinkle cinnamon on top. Rice and banana help stop diarrhea and return important nutrients lost.

Fever Reducing Treatment.

2 cups boiling water.
½ tsp. elder flower.
½ yarrow flowers.
½ peppermint leaves.
½ hyssop leaves.
Mix all ingredients and steep for 15 minutes, strain herbs. Give your child as much tea as possible. If he or she does not like the taste, mix it with fruit juice.

Food Allergy Treatment.   (See also Stomach Problems)

2 cups of water.
½ tsp. echinacea root.
½ tsp. marshmallow root.
1 tsp. chamomile flowers.
½ tsp. peppermint leaves.
1/4 tsp ginger rhizome.
Mix water, echinacea, and marshmallow roots, simmer for 5 minutes then add the rest of the ingredients and steep for 15 minutes. Strain and give 2 cups a day.

Attention Deficit Disorder (ADD)

ADD is the fastest growing childhood disorder in the United States. Almost 10% of school age children are suffering from this condition and the number keep growing every year. It affects boys more than girls and it causes a variety of learning and behavioral problems.

The reasons for this disorder are not yet clear. What's clear to me is that the treatments administered to children suffering from ADD is inadequate. Using drugs may be illegal but still doctors prescribe Ritalin and amphetamines. This does not address the problem and cause serious side effects, not to mention that these drugs are a form of "speed." Researchers discovered that Ritalin has many serious long term effects. Some of them are: decreased appetite, weight loss, insomnia, slowed growth, increased heart rate, increased blood pressure, increased irritability and the possibility of developing Parkinson's disease. Some reports have compared Ritalin to cocaine.

ADD is an imbalance in the brain. This disease is another reason to remove chemicals from our life. Our children are being bombarded with synthetic substances and chemicals: pesticides, mercury, lead, food additives, artificial sweeteners, vaccines, antibiotics and allergenic foods. It has been proven that these chemicals have a major impact in the development of brain cells and when combined they produce devastating effects.

The removal of these toxins is a must for a child suffering ADD and a common sense idea tells me that loading a child with potent drugs is not the best course of action. Herbs can relax and calm at first and in the long run they can improve brain function and neurotransmitter production. Other herbs can protect, detoxify and heal the nervous system. All this without side effects.

*California Poppy is a gentle sedative that relieves psychological and emotional disturbances in kids. It soothes and balances an overactive nervous system. It reduces anxiety and tension in overactive cases and decreases spasms. It is effective for difficulty in falling asleep or frequent regular waking.

*Grape Seed Extract contains bioflavonoids with the most potent antioxidant effects known. It is able to cross the blood brain barrier and directly protect the brain against a wide variety of toxins and damaging free radicals. It improves brain blood flow and strengthens brain capillaries.

*Oats are nutrients for the nervous system and a tonic for mental stress they improve mental concentration and focus.

*St. John's Wort is the herb of choice for kids suffering from ADD and/or hyperactivity. It calms the nervous system and regulates attention and anger.

*Valerian reduces restlessness and improves sleep with its relaxing and sedating properties. It creates improvements in learning skills and lessens aggressive behavior. It should be taken for four weeks to improve sleep and mood.

Hyperactivity Remedy.

> 1 tsp. Valerian rhizome tincture.
> ½ tsp. catnip leaves tincture.
> ½ tsp. passionflower leaves tincture.
> 1/4 tsp. peppermint leaves tincture.
> Mix all ingredients and give half a dropperfull 4 times a day.

*A change in the diet for a child with ADD is a must. Preservatives, artificial colors and artificial flavors are all chemicals that have a tremendous impact on the brain. In this section you'll find a list of all the foods that a child with ADD should and should not eat.

*Include fresh fruits and vegetables in their diets.

*Breads, crackers and cereals containing only rice and oats are needed for proper brain activity.

*Tuna, salmon and herring are important sources of docosahexaenoic acid (DHA) and essential fatty acid for brain development. This nutrient is often deficient in children with ADD.

*Foods rich in protein are needed to provide amino acids to the body.

*Limit the intake of dairy products especially if you notice behavioral changes when consumed.

*Remove completely all foods containing refined sugars, junk food, prepared frozen foods, foods that contain artificial flavors, artificial colors, monosodium glutamate, yeast, and/or preservatives.

*Remove natural foods that contain salicylates, like almonds, apples, apricots, all berries, cherries, cucumbers, currants, oranges, peaches, peppers, plums, prunes and tomatoes.

*Do not give any of the followings: apple cider vinegar, bacon, butter, candy, catsup, chocolate, colored cheeses, chili sauce, corn, ham, hotdogs, luncheon meat, margarine, meatloaf, milk, mustard, pork, salami, salt, soy sauce, sausage, tea, and wheat.

*Chemicals in perfumes, antacid tablets, and commercial toothpaste are very damaging for kids with ADD. Use a natural toothpaste from a health store.

Thrush infection.

Thrush is an infection that affects babies and young children. It causes white spots form in the mouth and it causes fever and indigestion. Antibiotics cause adverse reaction since this is yeast infection. Research done in Germany, England and Hungary have shown that many herbs inhibit this and other kinds of Candida bacteria.

Essential oils made out of the following herbs are used in Europe. Clove, tea tree, lavender, chamomile and garlic. All of these herbs combat the thrush infection.

Thrush fighting mixture.

    8 drops lavender essential oil.
    8 drops tea tree essential oil.
    2 tbsp. vegetable oil.
    Mix all ingredients and apply inside the baby's mouth using a cotton ball or a clean finger. If the baby is breast-feeding, put some oil several times a day over your nipples. This will prevent the back and forth infection between mother and child.

Ear infection:

The human ear is composed of the inner ear, middle ear, and the outer ear. Ear infection can attack any of these parts and one part can usually infect the others. External otitis affects the outer ear. It sometimes comes after a cold or flu or some other kind of upper respiratory infection. The area from the eardrum to the outer part becomes inflamed and is very painful. Sometimes a fever may be developed. Otitis media affects the area inside the eardrum and all the small bones. The air pressure is regulated in this area by the auditory tube running from the ear to the back of the nasal cavity. When bacteria or a virus gets in this area, the different parts become inflamed with fluid causing pressure and extremely sharp pain in the ear and can cause fever. If the infection is not controlled, it can result in eardrum perforation letting all pressure out and relieving pain, but a perforated eardrum means loss of hearing and fluid discharge. This kind of ear infection is very common in infants due to the position of the baby while feeding allowing milk bacteria to grow in the auditory tube.

We recommend

* Use Colloidal silver, as an ear wash, it can be taken orally too. This is a natural antibiotic.

* Take Vitamin C to help boost the immune system and fight infection.

* Zinc is also helpful in reducing ear infection.

* If the infection has just begun take echinacea (alcohol free).

* Mix lobelia and garlic oil or olive oil, place a few drops in the ear and plug it with cotton this will help with pain.

Make a tea mixing:
1 tsp. echinacea root.
1 tsp. licorice root.
2 tsp. ginkgo biloba leaves.
1 tsp. white willow bark.
1 tsp. ginger root.
3 cups of water.
Boil all ingredients for 15 minutes and take 1 cup a day.

Make a tea mixing:
1 tsp. black cohosh root.
1 tsp. kava kava root.
1 tsp. pulsatilla.
3 cups of water.
Boil for 15 minutes and take 20 teaspoons during the course of the day.

Ear Infection killer wash

16 ounces isopropyl alcohol
4 Tablespoons Boric Acid Powder
16 drops Gentian Violet Solution 1%
Mix altogether in a bottle (a hair dye type bottle is the best). Be very careful the gentian violet stains. Not so bad once it's mixed with the alcohol & boric acid but by itself it stains so when mixing together put gloves on.

* If the ear is red, hot and painful especially after exposure to cold temperature, use Aconite, this homeopathic remedy is excellent for ear infection.

* If the cheek of the same side of the ear affected is red and the person is unable to tolerate the pain then take chamomilla.

* If the area is overwhelmed with a pulsating pain and sensitive to touch, take hepar sulph.

Chickenpox:

Chickenpox is a very common and highly contagious viral infection disease. Newborns and adults may experience more severe symptoms than children who are at risk before the age of ten. Vaccinations have reduced its incidence. The symptoms for chickenpox fever, fatigue, itchy rash and loss of appetite do not appear until the infectious stage has begun.

This virus is transmitted by air (coughing and sneezing) or physical contact with a sick person. One or two days later pimple like eruptions appear on the body. They are filled with fluid and look like blisters, then they crust over. During this period itching can be very annoying but scratching can lead to infection and scarring.

Most of us are infected with this disease once in our lives. After the first exposure to the virus the body builds up immunity in the form of antibodies that recognize the disease and kills the virus before it can infect us again.

Chickenpox normally starts and finishes in about two weeks but people with weak immune systems or newborns can have very serious complications and if infected prenatally there is a risk of birth defects.

One of the factors that influence the chances of coming down with childhood diseases is the immune system. Some children seem to always catch something; flu, colds, stomach upsets, while others almost never get sick. The reason is that some kids have a stronger immune system then others. There are many things a parent can do to prevent instead of treating. Either way, you will find that herbs can help boost the immune system and cure diseases.

We all know that antibiotics have some side effects and as we have said before, giving antibiotics to a child from a very early age is not advisable because the viruses can develop resistance to the medicine which means that ever more powerful antibiotics have to be used in order to treat the problem and who would want a son or daughter to go through that. For this reason, we are going to show you how to make your own natural antibiotics for children.

We recommend

*Use Catnip tea sweetened with molasses. It reduces fever.

Make a tea with:
2 tbs. of queen of the meadow.
1 tsp. of coltsfoot leaves.
2 tsp. of marigold flowers.
2 cups of boiling water.
In a nonmetallic pot mix all ingredients and let sit for 20 minutes.
Take one cup a day.

Mix 2 tbs. marigold flowers.
     1 tsp. witch hazel leaves.
     1 cup of water.
Let them sit over night. Apply on rash as needed. It will relieve the itch of chickenpox.

*Some very useful homeopathic remedies are: Antimonium crudum, antimonium tartaricum, Pulsatilla, sulphur and rhus tox.

*Some very powerful herbs are: St. John's Wort, pau d'arco, ginger, burdock root, echinacea and goldenseal.

*Drink lots of water to prevent dehydration. Also drink fresh juices.

*Fill the bath tub with cool water, add ginger to it and take a 30 minute bath. This helps stop the itching.

TIP: Do not give aspirin to a child who has developed a fever.
It risks contracting Reye's syndrome, a dangerous and for some, fatal disease.

*Stay indoors with lights dimmed. Do not use bright lights or sunlight.

*Take baths with cornstarch or oatmeal (uncooked).

*Take Vitamin C with bioflavonoids. This will boost the immune system and keep fever low.

*People who had chickenpox and develop the symptoms again in adulthood may have a resurface of the virus which can lie dormant for many years in adults. This second infection is called Shingles.

Childhood disease remedy.

1 tsp. burdock root.
½ tsp. bupleurum root.
1 tsp. catnip leaves.
1 tsp. lemon balm leaves.
1 tsp. mullein leaves.
1 tsp. elder flowers.
½ tsp. yarrow flowers.
½ tsp. peppermint leaves.
1 liter of water.
Mix burdock, bupleurum and water and simmer for 5 minutes, remove from heat and add the rest of the herbs and steep for 20 minutes. Strain and drink 2 cups a day. For children that won't drink the remedy, mix it with fruit juice.

Treatment for blisters.

*Apply aloe vera juice to the blisters to improve healing.

*If the blister is infected, apply barberry.

*Bathe the blister with salty water. This will discourage the growth of bacteria thus preventing infection.

*For infected blisters, a poultice of roasted onions has been shown to improve the condition.

*Witch hazel applied to blisters will reduce pain, swelling and speed up healing.

*If the blisters break, clean the surrounding area and the open blisters with a few drops Roman chamomile and water.

Itching and blister remedy.

This remedy will stop the itching and speed up healing of blisters reducing the risk of infection.

2 tsp. burdock root.
2 tsp. calendula flowers.
2 tsp. lemon balm leaves.
6 drops of bergamot essential oil.
3 cups of water.
Simmer burdock in water for 5 minutes, remove from heat and add the rest of the herbs. Steep for 20 minutes and add the essential oil. Apply on the blisters by soaking and wringing a cotton cloth.

Immune system booster.

2 cups of boiling water.
1 tsp. echinacea root.
½ tsp. chamomile flowers.
½ tsp. shizandra berries if available.
½ tsp. of peppermint leaves.
Pour water over the herbs, steep for 20 minutes, strain. Give one cup a day at the first sign of illness.

Home made antibiotic. (For children)

2 cups water.
½ tsp. of echinacea root.
½ tsp. of licorice root.
½ cup of barberry bark. (Oregon grape root can be use instead)
2 cups of fresh apple juice.
Simmer herbs in water for 5 minutes, remove from heat, steep for 30 minutes, strain let it cool and add apple juice. Give one cup a day.

Fever:

Fever is an elevation in body temperature. It's the body's protective mechanism against infection. The elevation in temperature happens when our immune system is fighting off bacteria and viruses that could harm our body. Fever is our strongest weapon in the fight against infections or diseases.

Normal body temperature ranges from 97 to 99 degrees Fahrenheit but varies throughout the day. Usually it's lower in the early morning and higher in late afternoon. A fever is considered to be any temperature above 100 degrees Fahrenheit. One should be concerned when temperature rises above 102 degrees Fahrenheit for an adult and 103 degrees Fahrenheit for children.

Often, having a high temperature is helpful for the body; it's the way the body acts to destroy harmful microbes. In an adult temperature less than 103 degrees Fahrenheit encourage the body to create more immune cells. A fever of 104 or higher can be a risk for people with cardiac problems since it accelerates the heart beat making it work harder and can cause irregular rhythms, chest pain or even heart attack. When a person has had a fever of more than 106 degrees for a long period of time it can cause dehydration and brain damage.

Although vigorous exercise in which the muscles generate heat faster than the body can dissipate it can cause a temporary rise in temperature it is not considered fever.

We recommend:

* Drink as much water as you can in order to replace fluid loss. It will also help bring down body temperature.

* Rest as much as possible.

* Avoid sudden changes in atmospheric temperatures.

* Avoid eating solid foods until the fever is gone. You can replace the foods by drinking plenty of distilled water and/or juices.

* When you have fever do not take any supplement containing either iron or zinc. Taking iron causes great tension in a body that is fighting infection and zinc is not absorbed by the body when you have fever.

* Take cool baths. Fill a bath tub, submerge and lie down for approximately 5 minutes. Repeat as needed until the fever is down.

* If the fever does not exceed 102 degrees let it run its course. It helps the body fight infection and eliminate toxins.

* When a child has fever do not give them aspirin. Instead try to reduce the fever with cold baths.

* If a baby of 3 months or younger has 103 degrees or more, call your doctor. If a child with fever has also a stiff neck, swelling of the throat or disorientation, see a physician immediately as these symptoms may indicate meningitis.

* To reduce fever some beneficial herbs include Blackthorn, Echinacea, Fenugreek seed, Feverfew, Ginger and Poke root. Caution: Avoid Feverfew during pregnancy.

* Taking a tea or a hot steam bath made with Elderberry may help.

* If you develop an unusually high fever, sponge your face and forehead with lukewarm water. It will reduce the fever and you will feel more comfortable.

To reduce fever you can make this tea:
1 tsp. Echinacea root.
1 tsp. White willow root.
1 cup water.
Combine ingredients in a pan, cover and bring to a boil. Reduce heat and simmer for 30 minutes, cool and strain. Take half a cup up to 4 times a day.

Men's Health

For some reason men's health has been neglected in most books, as if men did not have concerns about their health or are not plagued by hundreds of diseases affecting only their gender. This section of the book deals with both specific and common illnesses that have affected males for hundreds of years. Even though modern medicine and conventional treatments have yet to find the cure for many conditions, herbs have been used effectively to fight against infections, infertility, impotence, hair loss, prostate problems, genital disorders and more.

Most physical problems in men are caused by hormonal imbalances, especially in the levels of testosterone (the male hormone). This hormone has many functions and it is responsible for the muscle formation, deep voice, hair and most of the characteristics that set men and women apart. Testosterone is produced in the testis and the adrenal glands. High levels of testosterone have been linked to prostate enlargement and over aggressive behavior. Low levels of testosterone are responsible for infertility, impotence, low sex drive and pour muscle development; that is why it is very important to maintain a healthy level of testosterone.

It's amazing that the female and male body need each other to evolve yet they are so different inside and out. Men need a completely different set of nutrients and remedies to maintain good health many drugs designed to treat hormonal problems can cause undesirable side effects.

Herbs have been used for thousands of years to treat male health problems and some plants have been nicknamed male plants, or male sex plants, for their incredible properties and fabulous effectiveness treating male conditions.

Remedies for men

Genital Infections.

Genital infections are usually sexually transmitted diseases (STDs). These reproductive system infections can cause all sorts of problems in the reproductive organs and if not treated properly can affect other organs and eventually impair general health. In North America more than 12 million cases a year are reported and it is estimated that many more are not reported simply because some STDs show no symptoms at all. Antibiotics have been used to control these bugs but the new arrivals like HIV and AIDS are not affected even by our most powerful drugs. Sexually Transmitted Diseases need professional treatment and early detection is very important to assure successful treatment and survival. However, herbs can help treat many irritations and infections on the genital area, for example, cases of rashes and infected wounds have been treated successfully with herbs.

Irritation and infection soak.

2 cups of water.
1 tsp. yarrow flowers.
1 tsp. lavender flowers.
1 tsp. goldenseal rhizome or Oregon grape root.
Mix herbs and pour boiling water over them, steep for 20 minutes. Strain and cool to a comfortable temperature. Soak affected area 2 time a day for five minutes.

Genital Infection and "jock Itch" Oil and Powder.

Jock itch is a fungal infection which irritates the area and produces an annoying itch and in some cases pain.

Infection affecting the genitals must be treated internally and externally below you will find some very powerful oil and powder remedies.

OIL.
1/8 tsp. lavender essential oil.
1/8 tsp. tea tree essential oil.
1 ounce vegetable oil.
Mix ingredients and apply directly to the infected are twice a day.

POWDER.
1 cup of cornstarch.
10 drops lavender essential oil.
10 drops tea tree essential oil.
10 drops goldenseal extract.
Mix ingredients inside of a self-sealing bag and shake well, breaking up the lumps of oil until smooth. Store the mixture for 3 days shaking every day for 2 minutes. Apply on the area once or twice a day. TIP: This powder is great for Athlete's foot too.

Follow the instructions below to prepare an Infection Treatment Extract. It also boosts the immune system.

Infection Treatment Extract.

½ ounce echinacea root tincture.
½ ounce goldenseal root tincture.
½ ounce pau d'arco bark tincture.
Mix all ingredients and take 15 drops 5 times a day for a week or until infection disappear.

Impotence.

Impotence is very common in men but it's a difficult subject to discuss. It is estimated that about 10 million men in the United States suffer from impotence. By age 65 a quarter of all men in North America are impotent. Impotence can be caused by low levels of testosterone, emotional mood, stress and fatigue overwork, and insufficient sleep also have an impact on testosterone level but not exclusively, poor circulation, prescription drugs for high blood pressure and recreational drugs like heroin can cause impotence as well.

TIP: Did you know that stress triggers the production of too much prolactin (a pituitary hormone) that causes impotence? If you drink beer at the end of a stressful day, you should know that the hops in beer increase prolactin too, the combination of stress and beer skyrocket the chances of developing impotence.   IN FACT: Beer disrupts hormonal balance, by rising prolactin and estrogen (female hormone), which in turn lowers testosterone (male hormone). This imbalance may be the cause for heavy beer drinking males to develop enlarged breasts and bellies.

TIP: Since stress causes impotence many doctors prescribe a pharmaceutical relaxant to reduce stress. But these drugs also reduce sexual desire and they interfere with performance.

* The herb Valerian is a natural relaxant that does not interfere with sexual functions.

* Skullcap and California Poppy reduce physical and emotional stress.

* Kava Kava and fresh oats relax the mind and body improving sexual performance.

Sex Drive Increaser (Aphrodisiac).

4 ounces sweet almond oil.
10 drops lavender essential oil. (Used to relax the muscles. Not an aphrodisiac)
10 drops sandalwood essential oil.
2 drops ylang-ylang essential oil.
2 drops vanilla essential oil.
1 drop cinnamon essential oil.
1 drop jasmine essential oil.
Mix all ingredients and use as aromatherapy to relax and increase sex drive.

Impotence Extract.

½ ounce ginseng root tincture.
½ ounce ginkgo leaves tincture.
½ ounce yohimbe bark tincture.
½ ounce fresh oat leaves tincture.
Mix all ingredients and take 30 drops 4 times a day for 2 months.

Fertility Formula.

1 ounce panax ginseng root tincture.
½ ounce fresh oats tincture.
½ ounce ashwaganda leaves tincture.
½ ounce raspberry leaves tincture.
Mix ingredients and take 20 drops 2 times a day.

Back Pain in men

About 80% of adults suffer from back pain at some time in their lives. Backaches are categorized as acute and chronic: acute pain is caused by movement or excessive use of the back which can injure the muscles, ligaments, bones or tendons.
Chronic pain is a recurring backache that restricts from normal movements or for no particular reason. It can also affect the tendons, ligaments, bones.

Problems with some organs can cause back pain as well, for example, kidney infection, prostate problems, bladder and even constipation can be felt on the lower back.

If you have back pain you can also feel muscle aches, locked areas in your back, stiff neck and your legs will ache as well.

Other causes of back pain can be poor postural habits, strains, microtrauma, muscle tension and nutritional deficiencies. When repeated episodes of injury are added to this mix, the discs become thin, deteriorated or ruptured. These events can also lead to arthritic related conditions. With nerves close by, swelling or compression in the spine often results in neuritis, lumbar neuralgia, or sciatica.

Herbal medicines are used in these conditions with far more safety than drugs.

We recommend

*Ask someone massage to the affected area with herbal oils using knuckles and increasing pressure slowly. After a few minutes you will feel less discomfort. This gets rid of tension and relaxes the muscles in that area.

*Every time you lift something, remember to bend your knees first, this will prevent your lower back from getting tense and causing damage to your spine and back muscles.

*Never twist while lifting. This can have bad effect on your vertebrates.

*Do not sit in couches, always sit in firm chairs supporting the lumbar area with a pillow. This will help you keep your waist and lower back in the proper position.

*Apply St. John's Wart directly to the back area. CAUTION: Do not expose yourself to the sun, this oil makes your skin very sensitive to the sun.

*Try to sleep with pillows supporting your back,and legs.

*Here are some homeopathic remedies that will help you with back pains: Cimicifuga, Kali carbonica. Lincopodium, Nux vomica and Arnica.

*Black Haw contains compounds very similar to the ones found in aspirin. It relieves spasms and neuralgia of back and neck, sciatica, leg cramps, tension headaches, wry neck.

*Boswellia is a strong anti-inflammatory. It reduces stiffness and pain. It has to be used for at least 4 weeks in chronic cases. It also improves circulation around ligaments, joints, and tendons.

*Jamaican Dogwood is a strong pain reliever, sedative and antispasmodic. It's very helpful for muscular back pain, asthma, insomnia, toothaches, and nervous conditions.

*Dong Quai has 1.5 times the analgesic activity of aspirin. It relieves back pain, cramping, muscular spasms and inflammation.

*The herb Cat's Claw grows in South America has been researched and proven to reduce inflammation while boosting the immune system. The studies also discovered that cat's claw contains anti arthritic compounds and is currently being used to treat people with rheumatoid arthritis.

*Take Vitamin E to protect and improve joint mobility.

*Bromelain comes from the stem of the pineapple, it contains anti-inflammatory blocks, reduces swelling, pain and damage to joints. A study done on 200 people showed a 75% reduction in inflammation, these results are better then the ones obtained using drugs. Finally, in the last few years Bromelain is being used in hospitals across U.S.

*Wild yam, is used for back pain characterized by sharp, knifelike sensations.

*Barberry is used for low back pain, often related to kidney weakness. Good for sciatica and neuralgia with radiating pain.

*Horsetail has high amounts of silica which is essential for bones and connective tissue.

*Eat alfalfa or take alfalfa extract in capsules. It contains all the necessary nutrients to alleviate back pain.

TIP: Make an home made ice pack by mixing 2 parts water and 1 part alcohol in a nylon bag and freezing it. The bag will be flexible thus molding to the body and it will not sweat.

*When pain hits suddenly, drink two large glasses of pure water. Dehydration can cause back pain.

*Several studies done in Scandinavia on smoking and non smoking twins have shown that smoking greatly aggravates problems in the disks. It's always advisable to quit smoking.

*Rhus Toxicodendrom is a homeopathic remedy that relieves stiffness.

Benign Prostatic Hypertrophy (B.P.H.):

The prostate is the male sex gland. It is the size of a chestnut and in the shape of a doughnut through which the urinary tract runs. The prostate is also in charge of discharging sperm during ejaculation. Semen is mainly made of prostatic fluid.

TIP: Did you know that sesame seeds are believed to enhance sexual vigor?

Benign prostatic hypertrophy is the gradual enlargement of the prostate. It's very a common problem for men more than fifty years of age and 75% of men more than seventy years of age suffer from it. It is caused by hormonal changes in the body as we age. Later in life men's production of dihydrotestosterone increases leading to an over production of prostate cells, this makes the prostate grow.

This condition develops symptoms such as, inability to empty the bladder, frequent urination, pain, burning, blood in the urine, difficulty starting and stopping urination. This disease can cause kidney damage due to the incomplete emptying of the bladder which causes pressure to the kidneys.

We recommend

TIP: Did you know that cranberry juice can prevent urinary tract infection? Which it has been linked to prostatitis.

* Saw Palmetto is an herb widely used in Germany for many years. It is the best long term treatment for benign prostatic hypertrophy (BPH) it reduces inflammation, pain, nocturnal urination, retention, difficulty starting urination, and dribbling. It's helpful for impotence,

and restores sex drive. It should be used for 6 to 12 months and is effective in 99% of patients.

* Goldenseal is a powerful antibiotic for effective treatment of prostatitis, killing most of the bacteria that cause the condition. It soothes and heals the urinary tract, helps shrink a swollen prostate.

* Lycopene is a bioflavonoid extracted from tomato. It reduces dribbling or frequency. It is a powerful antioxidant that prevents prostate cancer.

* Pollen (bee pollen) has shown remarkable success improving 80% of the cases and curing 40% of them within 6 months, especially if taken in the early stages. It shrinks enlarged prostates.

* Pygeum reduces size of the prostate in both acute and chronic prostatitis and in BPH, removes cholesterol from the prostate, and improves urinary flow.

* Tribulus is very helpful in treating prostatitis, prostate enlargement and semen production. It also improves impotence and sex drive.

TIP: Some over the counter cold or allergy medications can contribute to inflammation of the prostate and cause urine retention.

* Pumpkin seeds are used in prostate treatment for their essential fatty acids and their zinc contents. They reduce swelling. Pumpkin oil extract is easy to find in many health stores or eat 2 ounces a day of raw pumpkin seeds.

A tincture can be made by mixing:

1 ounce tincture of saw palmetto berries.
½ ounce tincture of nettle root.
½ ounce sarsaparilla root.
½ ounce pipsissewa leaves.
Use a dropper to take half three times a day.

* Pipsissewa is an herb from north America used to disinfect the urinary tract, good for bladder infection, prostatitis and prostate enlargement.

TIP: Did you know that vasectomy has been linked to prostate problems including cancer?

Mix ½ tsp. of lavender oil.
    ½ tsp. of rosemary oil.
      3 ounces of saint John's wort oil.
Rub the mixture under the scrotum once a day.

* Mix 1 tsp. of goldenseal root.
    1 tsp. of fringe tree bark.
    4 tsp. saw palmetto berries.
    3 cups of boiling water.
Steep for 45 minutes, strain, and drink 1 cup a day for a week, then reduce to 3 cups a week.

TIP: The drug leuprolide (Lupron) shrinks the prostate, but it causes impotence, low sex drive and hot flashes.

* Use horsetail combined with hydrangea if you see blood in the urine and have frequent urination.

* Siberian ginseng and Panax ginseng are tonics used in china for the male reproductive system and enlarged prostate.

* Drink 2 quarts of pure water a day. This helps clean the urinary tract and prevents kidney infection.

* Evening primrose has been successfully used to treat prostate problems.

* The aquatic plant Watercress helps fight urinary infections and prostate problems. The leaves should be eaten frequently to alleviate the problem.

Migraine:

Migraine is the term used to describe a severe pain in the head. This can be caused by the contraction or dilatation of blood vessels in the brain and the irregular nerve activity mainly in the meninges. Migraine is caused by the stimulation of the trigeminal nerve which release a substance inducing inflammation and also sends messages to pain receptors in the meninges.

People who suffer from migraines often are between the ages of 20 and 30. However, children can have migraines too but their symptoms are shown as colic, periodic abdominal pains, vomiting, dizziness and severe motion sickness. Then these symptoms will disappear, focusing in the exact problem, painful headaches. Almost every person who suffers from migraines will have some symptoms before having one.

There are five phases

1. The day before the person has a migraine there may be a very noticeable change in the mood or problems remembering things or an alteration in one or all of the five senses or he/she could have speech problems.

2. A moment before the migraine begins some people see flashes or experience numbness of the hands and mouth.

3. Once the migraine starts the pain could be overwhelming. It may be at one or both sides of the head. You can experience some nausea along with sensitivity in the neck and scalp.

4. The headaches will soon disappear including the nausea.

5. After these symptoms you may feel tired, without energy and will want to sleep.

A migraine can be due to allergies, constipation, stress, liver malfunction, too much or too little sleep, emotional changes, hormonal changes, suns glare, flashing lights, poor exercise, dental problems, low blood sugar and changes in the barometric pressure.

We recommend:

* Eat a diet that is low in carbohydrates and high in protein. Try to include in your diet almonds, watercress, parsley, fennel, garlic, cherries and pineapple.

* Avoid alcohol, processed meat (hot dogs), chocolates, aspirin, avocados, beer, bananas, canned fish, cabbage, eggplant, dairy products, potatoes, hard cheeses, tomatoes, wine, red plums, yeast, raspberries, salt, meat, cereal, grains, bread, fried foods and greasy foods.

* Do not miss any meal. Instead eat small, nutritious meals and have some snacks if needed.

* Take only hypoallergenic supplements.

* Get plenty of exercise.

* During the day massage your neck and the back of your head several times to relieve tension.

* Try to be always in a calm ambient, avoid strong odors and high altitudes.

* Do not smoke and do not allow people to smoke in front of you.

* Take a cup of strong coffee to relieve pain caused by migraine.

* To prevent or control the migraine supplements are needed such as:
Calcium + Magnesium. They help to regulate muscle tone and to transmit nerve impulses throughout the body and to the brain.

* Primrose oil has an anti-inflammatory agent that keeps the blood vessels from constricting.

* Multivitamin and mineral formulas are necessary daily to complement the nutrients we do not include in our diet.

* Rutin removes toxic metals which may cause migraines.

* Garlic is a potent detoxifier.

* Vitamin C with bioflavonoids helps in producing an anti stress adrenal hormone and enhances immunity.

* In addition are a variety of herbs that can help control and relieve migraines:

Cordyceps reduces anxiety and stress and at the same time promotes sleep.

Feverfew reduces discomfort and pain. Caution: Avoid during pregnancy.

* Gingko Biloba extract enhances cerebral circulation.

* Iris versicolor relieves pain and discomfort.

* To alleviate migraines massage one drop of peppermint oil into each temple.

* You can also drink one cup infusion of Hops or take ½ tsp. extract 3 times daily.

* At the first sign of a migraine take Black Willow, Jamaican Dogwood, Passion Flower, Valerian or Wood Betony to ease the pain.

* To ease pain, instead of taking pain killers that have serious side effects, try making these teas, are natural and have no side effects.
1 tsp. Feverfew leaves.
1 tsp. Peppermint leaves.
1 cup boiling water.
Mix all the herbs in a nonmetallic container and cover with the boiling water, steep for 30minutes, then strain. If you want, add honey for taste. Take one tbs. at a time. Throughout the day you should drink more than one cup of the tea.

Prostatitis:

The prostate is the male sex gland the size of a chestnut and in the shape of a doughnut through which the urinary tract runs. The prostate is also in charge of discharging sperm during ejaculation. Semen is mainly made of prostatic fluid.

Prostatitis is an inflammation in the prostate gland. This is a very common problem for men of all ages. Bacteria from different parts of the body infect the prostate and that causes prostatitis. Once infected the prostate swells restricting the flow of urine and causing urine retention. There are three types of prostatitis: acute infectious prostatitis, chronic infectious prostatitis and noninfectious prostatitis.

Acute infectious prostatitis is caused by bacteria and the main symptoms are pain while urinating, burning feeling while urinating, pain under the scrotum, feelings of full bladder, pus or blood in urine, frequent urination (specially during the night) and fever.

Chronic infectious prostatitis is also cause by bacteria but the symptoms are as painful as acute infectious prostatitis and include burning while urinating, frequent urination, urging of urinating even when the bladder has been empty, cloudy urine, blood in urine, an unpleasant odor in urine. This may affect the person several times and is a long term problem.

Noninfectious prostatitis is not due to bacteria and the real cause is unknown. The symptoms are the same as the others plus there is pain while ejaculating and under the nibble.

We recommend

TIP: Did you know that cranberry juice can prevent urinary tract infection which has been linked to prostatitis?

* Saw Palmetto it's a herb widely used in Germany for many years. It is the best long term treatment for benign prostatic hypertrophy BPH. It reduces inflammation, pain, nocturnal urination, retention, difficulty starting urination and dribbling. It's helpful for impotence and restores sex drive. It should be used for 6 to 12 months and is effective in 99% of patients.

* Goldenseal is a powerful antibiotic for effective treatment of prostatitis, killing most of the bacteria that cause this condition. It soothes and heals the urinary tract and helps shrink a swollen prostate.

* Lycopene is a bioflavovoid extracted from tomato. It reduces dribbling or frequency. It is a powerful antioxidant that prevents prostate cancer.

* Pollen (bee pollen) has shown remarkable success improving 80% of the cases and curing 40% of them within 6 months, especially if taken in the early stages. It shrinks enlarged prostates.

* Pygeum reduces size of the prostate in both acute and chronic prostatitis and in BPH, removes cholesterol from the prostate and improves urinary flow.

* Tribulus is very helpful in treating prostatitis, prostate enlargement and semen production and improves impotence and sex drive.

TIP: Some over the counter cold or allergy medications can contribute to inflaming the prostate and retaining urine.

* Pumpkin seeds are used in prostate treatment for their essential fatty acids and their zinc contents. They reduce swelling. Pumpkin oil extract is easy to find in many health stores or eat 2 ounces a day of raw pumpkin seeds.

* A tincture can be made by mixing:
    1 ounce tincture of saw palmetto berries.
    ½ ounce tincture of nettle root.
    ½ ounce sarsaparilla root.
    ½ ounce pipsissewa leaves.
Take half a dropperful three times a day.

* Pipsissewa is a herb from North America used to disinfect the urinary tract. It is good for bladder infection, prostatitis and prostate

enlargement.

TIP: Did you know that vasectomy has been linked to prostate problems including cancer?

* Mix ½ tsp. of lavender oil.
       ½ tsp. of rosemary oil.
       3 ounces of saint John's wort oil.
Rub the mixture under the scrotum once a day.

* Mix 1 tsp. of goldenseal root.
      1 tsp. of fringe tree bark.
      4 tsp. saw palmetto berries.
      3 cups of boiling water.
Steep for 45 minutes, strain and drink 1 cup a day for a week, then reduce to 3 cups a week.

TIP: The drug leuprolide (Lupron) shrinks the prostate, but it causes impotence, low sex drive and hot flashes.

* Use horsetail combined with hydrangea if you see blood in the urine and have frequent urination.

* Siberian ginseng is a tonic used in china for the male reproductive system.

* Drink 2 quarts of pure water a day as this help clean the urinary tract and prevents kidney infection.

Women's Health

The differences between the male and female body are obvious but their immune and hormonal systems are very far apart. Many of the conditions that affect women are hormonal in nature which makes them very annoying due to the wide array of symptoms. An imbalance in Estrogen, the principal female hormone, is one of the most common problems affecting women from PMS to menopause. Hormonal problems can cause miscarriages as well. Women's hormones and bodies change a great deal while pregnant, which brings a whole new set of problems. Also, the reproductive system of a woman goes through a variety of changes during the course of life.

For these reasons this book contains a special section for women covering common ailments and specific conditions that affect females. We should clarify that some illnesses are very hard to diagnose especially those that have to do with hormones, therefore, we strongly recommend that you visit your physician to determine what the problem is, and only then should you try a natural treatment approach.

If the condition is not life threatening or serious, then you can choose from the remedies we suggest. Fortunately, herbs can help control and bring back to balance the female systems. The best part is that they do it without side effects or long term consequences.

TIP: Nursing mothers sometimes develop a fungus infection called Candida infection of the nipples. This causes severe pain while feeding and could be more complicated if the baby develops Oral Thrush, a fungal infection of the mouth which causes mother and baby to reinfect each other.

TIP: Did you know that the herb Saw Palmetto helps increase breast size especially at puberty.

Endometriosis

Endometriosis occurs when tissue from the lining of the uterus (the endometrium) attaches itself elsewhere in the abdomen. This brings a wide array of problems especially before menstruation when the lining expands.

Endometriosis affects about 10% of women in the U.S. However European females rarely get this disease. It is very painful, cramps in the abdomen are quite common. Other symptoms are, intestinal gas, excessive menstrual bleeding, insomnia and depression. This disease can cause infertility.

The reason for this disorder is not clear but what we know is that excessive amount of estrogen has an impact on the severity of endometriosis.
The drugs usually prescribed for the disease causes vaginal dryness, low sex drive, and menopause symptoms. Herbs can offer some help without complications.

We recommend

* Burdock is one of the best herbs to clean the liver and as we know estrogen is excreted by the liver. An efficient liver will rid estrogen more quickly.

* To reduce bleeding, inflammation and cramps, use wild yam, primrose, and ginger. Since these symptoms are similar to the ones for PMS, use the remedies we suggest in the PMS section of this book.

Endometriosis Tea.

1 tsp. vitex berries.
1 tsp. echinacea root.
1 tsp. wild yam rhizome.
1 tsp. cramp bark.
½ tsp. horsetail stalks.
½ tsp. red raspberry.
½ tsp. motherwort.
1 quart water.

Mix herbs and water in a saucepan and boil. Simmer for 5 minutes and steep for another 10 minutes. Strain and drink 2 cups a day.

The herb vitex berry controls estrogen which is one of the causes of endometriosis. By controlling levels of estrogen, this herb helps reduce the symptoms.

To reduce the size of the uterus use raspberry extract. It has been used to reduce bleeding for hundreds of years.

Infertility

Infertility is usually referred to as the incapacity to conceive after a year or more of regular sexual activity during the time of ovulation. Infertility affects 6 million couples in the United States and finding the reason for infertility can be difficult. There are many conditions that can cause infertility, some of them require surgery to be corrected others are caused by hormonal imbalance. Herbs can help in almost all cases in which hormones are the reason for infertility. That's why you should first find out the cause of the infertility before choosing a specific herbal treatment.

Some of the causes of infertility are:

* Stress can prevent ovulation.

* Very athletic women, with very low body fat, stop ovulating. This is a common problem for professional athletes.

TIP: Did you know that some women develop antibodies to their partners' sperm, in effect becoming allergic to them?

* Some contraceptives disrupted the hormonal balance causing infertility.

* Women with depress immune systems often are unable to become pregnant or they usually miscarry early in the pregnancy.

* Irregular menstrual cycles can make it very hard for some women to become pregnant.

*Endometriosis causes infertility. See endometriosis .

We recommend

* A study done in United States showed that women suffering from stress were able to become pregnant after learning relaxation techniques. See stress in this book.

* Studies on don quai show that it helps ovaries function better and it restores normal cycles.

* The herb vitex has been researched in Germany. That research has shown that vitex increases the levels of three hormones: progesterone, prolactin and luteinizing hormone (LH). These hormones help women become pregnant, sustain pregnancy and produce milk.

* Wild yam helps the uterus during pregnancy thus reducing the chances of miscarriage.

Fertility Herbal Treatment.

1 tsp. don quai root.
1 tsp. siberian ginseng root.
1 tsp. vitex berries.
1 tsp. motherwort leaves.
1 tsp. cramp bark.
1 tsp. wild yam rhizome.
1 quart water.
Mix herbs and simmer for 10 minutes. Steep for 10 minutes, strain and drink 2 cups a day.

* If you are not allergic to bee pollen, include it in your diet. Royal jelly is very helpful as well.

TIP: Did you know that alcohol prevents implantation of the fertilized egg in women?

Irregular Menstruation and hormonal Tonic.

1 tsp. vitex berries.
1 tsp. don quai root.
1 tsp. licorice root.
½ tsp. motherwort leaves.
½ tsp. siberian ginseng root.
1 quart of water.
Mix all ingredients, simmer for 10 minutes and steep for 20 minutes. Strain and drink 1 cup a day during menstruation until ovulation. If you are not menstruating, drink throughout the month.

TIP: Did you know that Ulcer medications cimetidine (Tagamet) and ranitidine (Zantac) may decrease the sperm count in some men and even produce impotence?

Miscarriage Prevention.

1 tsp. false unicorn root.
1 tsp. cramp bark.
½ tsp. red raspberry leaves.
½ tsp. wild yam root.
3 cups water.
Boil water and herbs and simmer for 10 minutes. Steep for 10 minutes, strain and drink 8 cups during the course of a day. If you find this to be too much liquid, you can use these herbs in a tincture and take 2 drops each false unicorn and cramp bark, 1 drop each red raspberry and wild yam 4 times a day.

Vaginal Infections.

Douche for vaginal infections.

3 drops lavender essential oil.
3 tea tree essential oil.
3 cups of warm water.
3 tbs.. of yogurt.
Mix ingredients in a douche bag. Use as needed for a week.

Vaginal infection tea.

1 tsp. cramp bark.
1 tsp. burdock root.
1 tsp. echinacea root.

1 tsp. oregon grape root.
1 tsp. vitex seeds.
1 quart of water.
Mix all herbs and simmer for 10 minutes, remove from heat and steep for 15 minutes. Strain and drink 3 cups a day.

* Barberry has remarkable infection fighting properties.

* Goldenseal used as an external topic or vaginal suppository is very helpful for all types of infections.

* Colloidal silver is a natural antibiotic that kills many types of bacteria.

* Tea tree oil is good for vaginitis. A cream made with tea tree oil is very effective against fungal infections, herpes blisters, wartsand other types of infections. A tea tree oil suppository has been used for years to fight yeast infections.

TIP: Did you know that eating yogurt and applying yogurt directly to the vagina, helps fight infections and relieves inflammation?

* Peel and blend 4 pieces of garlic and 1 cup of apple cider vinegar and 2 cups of warm water. Strain and wash vagina with the liquid.

Fibrocystic breast:

Fibrocystic breast is a condition that develops when fluid is not being evacuated fast enough from the breast causing cysts to form in them. These lumps move around the breast, grow and shrink, but they are benign.

Normally the fluids in the breast are transported out by the lymphatic system. But if there is too much fluid some may get deposited in different areas of the breast. Tissue grows around them creating these lumps. Like we said before these cysts are harmless but they should be monitored and a woman should check her breasts frequently in order to find and control the cysts. Frequent mammograms are recommended too.

Discomfort, tenderness, and noticeable growth are normal especially around menstrual periods when estrogen levels change. The cysts may disappear after the monthly period. However if the lump is hard and does not move freely and does not go away, check with a doctor immediately.

We recommend

TIP: Did you know that the herb Saw Palmetto helps increase breast size especially at puberty?

* Coenzyme Q10 is very important to remove toxins from the body and help control fibrocystic breasts.

* In many studies Primrose oil has been shown to reduce size of lumps.

* Take vitamin E. It's an antioxidant that protects breast tissue against fibrocystic breasts.

* Vitamin B6 manages fluids and hormone levels.

* The herb astragalus increases circulation to the surface of the skin helping to evacuate toxins.

* Black cohosh regulates menstrual periods and hormone levels reducing the chance of developing fibrocystic breasts.

* Castor oil is used frequently to shrink the size of cysts if used during several months.

* Burdock is very helpful in draining fluid and removing toxins reducing fibrocystic breasts.

* Poke root cleans the lymphatic fluid and clears abscesses present in fibrocystic breasts.

* Chasteberry balances estrogen helping reduce the development of cysts if used for several months.

* Examine your breast once a month. This can help detect early tumors or fibrocystic breasts.

* Don't drink coffee, regular tea, colas or chocolate and any foods that contain caffeine as it has been proven to increase fibrocystic breasts.

Breast Cyst tea.

1 tsp. burdock root.
1 tsp. mullein leaves.
1 tsp. dandelion root.
1/2 tsp. prickly ash bark.
1/2 tsp. cleavers leaves.
1 quart water.
Mix ingredients and drink 2 cups a day.

Breast compress.

1/2 tsp. calendula flowers tincture.
10 drops lavender essential oil.
3 drops ginger essential oil.
3 drops chamomile essential oil.
1 cup warm water.

1 cotton cloth.
Mix all ingredients, soak rag in the solution and place it over the area where the cysts are for 5 minutes, then repeat.

Frigidity:

Frigidity is mostly used to describe a sexual dysfunction in women and is the inability to experience pleasure from sexual intercourse. It is characterized by a lack of sexual desire and responsiveness due to traumatic sexual experience or other unpleasant episodes during childhood or as an adolescent. It is caused by psychological origin, stemming from fear, anxiety, guilt, depression, problems with the partner and/or feelings of inferiority.

Some women find intercourse painful due to poor lubrication, inadequate stimulation, some illness or infection or it can be related to other physical causes. The pain that these women experience causes them to shrink and fear from sexual contact with the partner. Vitamin deficiency can cause a deficiency in estrogen levels and lead to improper lubrication. Low sexual desire can also be due to a chronic illness, the use of some medications, low testosterone levels or a certain medical condition.

We recommend:

* Make sure that in your diet you are including a good quantity of alfalfa sprouts, avocados, eggs that come fresh from hens (avoid the ones stored cold in the supermarket), olive oil, pumpkin seeds, other seeds and nuts, soy and sesame oil and wheat.

* Avoid red meat, poultry and products containing sugar.

* Avoid smoggy conditions. Smog is highly toxic and dangerous and affects the entire immune function and hormonal activity in the body.

* Also herbs can help cope with the problem. Here are the most common:

Chives contain minerals required for the creation of sex hormones.

Damiana the " woman's sexuality herb", is the most popular aphrodisiac plant. This plant contains alkaloids that stimulate the nerves and organs. It's perfect for supporting the sexual organs and enhancing sexual pleasure.

Kava kava helps deal with anxiety and nervousness. Caution: Not recommended for pregnant women or nursing mothers. It should not be taken together with alcohol, barbiturates, antidepressants, antipsycotic drugs or any other substance that acts upon the central nervous system.

Wild yam contains a natural steroid that gives vigor to lovemaking and rejuvenates.

There are other great herbs used in promoting energy and sexuality such as: fo-ti, gotu kola, sarsaparrilla and saw palmetto.

* Some supplements can help such as:

Kelp: 2,000-2,500 mg daily; it's a good source of iodine and other important minerals.

Vitamin B complex: 100 mg of each major B vitamin twice daily; aids in reducing anxiety and calms the nervous system.

Vitamin E: Start taking 200-400 IU daily and increase slowly to 1,600 IU daily; it's necessary for the good functioning of the reproductive system and glands. Use the d-alphatocopherol form.

Menopause

Menopause is not a disease, but a new phase in an older woman's life, it usually causes ovulation to cease and consequently menstruation stops. This natural progression in life starts many years before menopause symptoms actually begin to show. Hormone levels can fluctuate for several years before eventually becoming so low that the endometrium stays thin and does not bleed. Normally the ovaries start to slow the production of hormones like estrogen, testosterone and progesterone. Although estrogen is an important sex and reproductive hormone, it is also present in many non reproductive organs and the body uses estrogen for many other functions, like bone formation, heart, liver breast and bladder function, it is need as well to keep the skin moist and healthy, and to regulate body temperature.

Low estrogen levels causes changes in collagen production, affecting hair, nails, skin and tendons. The skin may become dryer, thinner, less elastic, more prone to bruising and skin itching may occur.
The main symptoms of menopause are Hot flushes, Night sweats, Palpitations, Insomnia, Joint aches, Headaches, Vaginal dryness.
On the long run the shortage of estrogen contributes to developing heart disease, cardiovascular problems, osteoporosis, tooth decay, and a variety of vaginal complications.

The average age of the natural menopause is 51 years, but can occur much earlier or later. Menopause occurring before the age of 45 is called early menopause and before the age of 40 is premature menopause. Perimenopause is the stage from the beginning of menopausal symptoms to the postmenopause.

Postmenopause is the time following the last period, and is usually defined as more than 12 months with no periods in someone with intact ovaries, or immediately following surgery if the ovaries have been removed.

Complete symptom list:

Hot Flashes:
Our body's thermostat is located in the hypothalamus are of the brain, which stops working properly if level of estrogen are not sufficient. This will cause you to experience extremely hot or cold sensations; sometimes you could feel so hot that you would want to strip your close in public while other people feel very comfortable with the temperature and other times you could feel shivering cold in 90 degrees F.

Sleep Problems:
It is not certain if estrogen have an effect on sleeping patterns, however other symptoms caused by estrogen deficiency could be culprit of sleep problems during and after menopause, irritability, hot flashes during the night. Hormone replacement has shown to improve insomnia and sleeping problems, but this could be related to the reduction of

hot flushes, mood swings and irritability all of which are helped by increasing levels of estrogen.

Vaginal Dryness:
And inadequate vaginal lubrication can be a very disturbing for most women due to the pain, discomfort and sometimes bleeding experienced during sexual intercourse. Without estrogen

Aches and Pains:
One peculiar symptom of menopause is an increase in frequency of normal aches, such as, headaches, neck, joint and back pains are most common.

Bladder Problems:
Most women going through menopause complain of the following bladder problems, bladder infection, low bladder capacity, inability to contain urine, frequent urination. These problems start when bladder tissue becomes to be deprived of estrogen.

Skin Problems:
Our skin and collagen fibers are very sensitive to levels of estrogen, a hormone deficiency causes, dry, thinner and aging looking skin, irritation, and wrinkles.

Emotions:
Irritability, depression, personality changes and anxiety are very common during depression; these changes can carry a loss of sexual desire. Although these problems are related to the shortage of estrogen, some may be caused by the inability to cope with the psychological impact caused by all the other symptoms. Added to all this is the fact that in many cases women going through menopause might also be under a number of other stressful situations during this period. Things like teenage children, children moving out, aging parents and spouse's mid-life crisis can also influence in the state of mind of menopausal women.

Many of the symptoms and discomforts experienced during menopause can be relieved by using natural home remedies, things like changing your diet and using some very specific herbs have shown remarkable improvements in women going through menopause.

We recommend

* To increase your levels of estrogen try increasing your consumption of plants which contain estrogenic substances:
Alfalfa, soybeans, soy sprouts, crushed flaxseeds, garlic, green beans, sesame seeds, wheat, yams, pumpkin seeds, cucumbers, corn, apples, anise seeds, cabbage, beets, olive oil, olives, papaya, oats, peas, sunflower seeds, are all important sources of natural estrogens and as you can imagine they are loaded with vitamins, fiber and minerals essential not only for menopause, but to maintain an overall good health.

* To reduce hot flashes:
Drink 8 glasses of steam-distilled water.
Take 800 mg. of evening primrose oil, three times a day.
Take 300 IU. of vitamin E a day.

Hot Flashes Reducing tincture.
2 teaspoons of cohosh root tincture.
1 teaspoon of don quai root tincture.
1 teaspoon of sarsaparilla tincture.
1 teaspoon of licorice root tincture.
1 teaspoon of chaste tree tincture.
1 teaspoon ginseng root tincture.
Mix all the ingredients and take 3 dropperfuls a day.

Toner for Dry Skin.
Toners are used to improve the appearance of the skin, to soothe and to nourish. Men can use toners as aftershaves.
2 ounces aloe vera gel.
2 ounces orange-blossom water.
1 tsp. wine vinegar.
6 drops rose geranium essential oil.
4 drops sandalwood essential oil.
1 drop chamomile essential oil. *
800 UI vitamin E oil. (Puncture a gel capsule with a needle)

Cream for Dry Skin.
3/4 ounces beeswax, shaved. (do not use paraffin)
1 cup vegetable oil.
1 cup of distilled water.
800 IU vitamin E (from a liquid gel)
24 drops rose geranium essential oil.
Heat beeswax and oil in a pot until beeswax melts (it should be warm enough to the touch but without discomfort). In a separate pot heat water until is warm to the touch. Remove the center part of your blender's lid and pour the water in. Turn the blender on high speed and slowly but steadily add the oil and wax mixture. The whole concoction should begin to solidify. Keep adding oil until the mixture does not take any more. Turn off the blender and using a spatula, place the cream in a wide mouthed container.

*   Take 50mcg. of selenium 2,000 mg of vitamin C and 10 mg of beta-carotene, once a day to improve skin and help with vaginal dryness.

Vaginal Dryness lotion
1 ounce of almond oil.
2 drops of geranium essential oil.
One capsule of 1,000 IU of Vitamin E.
Mix all the ingredients and apply inside and outside the vagina twice a day.

Memory and Energy Tea
1 teaspoon of ginkgo biloba.
2 teaspoon of ginseng root.
1 teaspoon of royal jelly.
Mix the herb and add 1 liter of boiling water, steep for 15 minutes, add royal jelly and drink 2 cups a day.

* Take 1,000 mg of calcium, 25 mg of silica, 10 mcg of vitamin K, and 500mg of magnesium at bedtime to improve joint and bone strength.

* To improve anxiety and insomnia mix the following ingredients:
  1 tsp. chamomile flowers.
  1 tsp. hops.
  1 tsp. valerian root.
  1 cup of boiling water.
Steep for 45 minutes, strain and drink 1 hour before bedtime.

* Skullcap relieves insomnia caused by anxiety, worry or pain.

Migraine:

Migraine occurs most often in women due to fluctuations in the level of the hormone estrogen, that's the reason why women get migraines around the time of menstruation when estrogen levels are low.

During pregnancy is also common to suffer migraines especially during early pregnancy. The cause may be hormonal but the headache can be due to excess tension too.

Migraine is the term used to describe a severe pain in the head. This can be caused by the contraction or dilatation of blood vessels in the brain and the irregular nerve activity mainly in the meninges. Migraine is caused by the stimulation of the trigeminal nerve which release a substance inducing inflammation and also sends messages to pain receptors in the meninges.

People who suffer from migraines often are between the ages of 20 and 30. However, children can have migraines too but their symptoms are shown as colic, periodic abdominal pains, vomiting, dizziness and severe motion sickness. Then these symptoms will disappear, focusing in the exact problem, painful headaches. Almost every person who suffers from migraines will have some symptoms before having one.

There are five phases

1. The day before the person has a migraine there may be a very noticeable change in the mood or problems remembering things or an alteration in one or all of the five senses or he/she could have speech problems.

2. A moment before the migraine begins some people see flashes or experience numbness of the hands and mouth.

3. Once the migraine starts the pain could be overwhelming. It may be at one or both sides of the head. You can experience some nausea along with sensitivity in the neck and scalp.

4. The headaches will soon disappear including the nausea.

5. After these symptoms you may feel tired, without energy and will want to sleep.

A migraine can be due to allergies, constipation, stress, liver malfunction, too much or too little sleep, emotional changes, hormonal changes, suns glare, flashing lights, poor exercise, dental problems, low blood sugar and changes in the barometric pressure.

We recommend:

* Eat a diet that is low in carbohydrates and high in protein. Try to include in your diet almonds, watercress, parsley, fennel, garlic, cherries and pineapple.

* Avoid alcohol, processed meat (hot dogs), chocolates, aspirin, avocados, beer, bananas, canned fish, cabbage, eggplant, dairy products, potatoes, hard cheeses, tomatoes, wine, red plums, yeast, raspberries, salt, meat, cereal, grains, bread, fried foods and greasy foods.

* Do not miss any meal. Instead eat small, nutritious meals and have some snacks if needed.

* Take only hypoallergenic supplements.

* Get plenty of exercise.

* During the day massage your neck and the back of your head several times to relieve tension.

* Try to be always in a calm ambient, avoid strong odors and high altitudes.

* Do not smoke and do not allow people to smoke in front of you.

* Take a cup of strong coffee to relieve pain caused by migraine.

* To prevent or control the migraine supplements are needed such as:
Calcium + Magnesium. They help to regulate muscle tone and to transmit nerve impulses throughout the body and to the brain.

* Primrose oil has an anti-inflammatory agent that keeps the blood vessels from constricting.

* Multivitamin and mineral formulas are necessary daily to complement the nutrients we do not include in our diet.

* Rutin removes toxic metals which may cause migraines.

* Garlic is a potent detoxifier.

* Vitamin C with bioflavonoids helps in producing an anti stress adrenal hormone and enhances immunity.

* In addition are a variety of herbs that can help control and relieve migraines:

Cordyceps reduces anxiety and stress and at the same time promotes sleep.

Feverfew reduces discomfort and pain. Caution: Avoid during pregnancy.

* Gingko Biloba extract enhances cerebral circulation.

* Iris versicolor relieves pain and discomfort.

* To alleviate migraines massage one drop of peppermint oil into each temple.

* You can also drink one cup infusion of Hops or take ½ tsp. extract 3 times daily.

* At the first sign of a migraine take Black Willow, Jamaican Dogwood, Passion Flower, Valerian or Wood Betony to ease the pain.

* To ease pain, instead of taking pain killers that have serious side effects, try making these teas, are natural and have no side effects.
1 tsp. Feverfew leaves.
1 tsp. Peppermint leaves.
1 cup boiling water.
Mix all the herbs in a nonmetallic container and cover with the boiling water, steep for 30minutes, then strain. If you want, add honey for taste. Take one tbs. at a time. Throughout the day you should drink more than one cup of the tea.

P.M.S. (Prementrual Syndrome):

Prementrual syndrome is the most common gynecological complaint of women and it affects about 60% of them. The symptoms appear one or two weeks before menstruation starts, and they include: abdominal bloating and cramps, acne, anxiety, breast tenderness and swelling and mood changes.

During menstruation there is an imbalance in hormones and brain activity and it is believed that too much estrogen, uneven levels of progesterone and an inability to cope with hormone changes are the main causes of PMS. But the real reason as to why this condition affects so many women is unknown.

About 5% of women suffer such severe complications that they are incapable of functioning normally during this period. Others claim symptoms interfere with their daily activities.

Using herbs we can return hormone levels to their normal level and proper diet can help reduce many of the symptoms. The final result is a body that is back in balance without using drugs and without experiencing any side effects.

We recommend

* Take magnesium 1,000 mg. a day. Deficiencies have been linked to PMS.

* Take calcium 1,500 mg. a day to help reduce some symptoms.

* Take Vitamin B6 to reduce water retention and increase blood circulation to the female organs.

* Take Vitamin E to help reduce breast soreness.

TIP: Did you know that caffeine makes the changes of suffering from severe PMS symptoms 4 times greater?

* Black cohosh relieves premenstrual tension, menstrual cramps and water retention and helps control mood changes.

* Dandelion root is a very powerful diuretic that helps evacuate excess water and bloating but is safer then commercial diuretics because it does not deplete potassium. Another important quality is that it helps the liver discard estrogen thus relieving PMS.

* Dong Quai reduces cramps, pain and mood changes and regulates phytoestrogen leveling the hormones.

* Maca regulates hormones according to the body's need. It reduces acne occurrences and contains minerals and vitamins needed during PMS.

* Wild yam regulates levels of estrogen and progesterone. It relaxes the muscles and nerves.

* Studies have shown that Chaste tree regulates hormonal changes, reduces anxiety, mood changes and water retention and breast pain.

Mix the following ingredients:
    1 tsp. of black cohosh root.
    1 tsp. of passionflower.
    1 tsp. of oregon grape root.
    1 tsp. white willow bark.
    2 cup of water.
Boil for 30 minutes, strain, take one tbsp. per hour.

Make a tea mixing:
    1 tsp. black haw.
    1 tsp. licorice root.
    1 tsp. evening primrose.
    1 tsp. milk thistle.
    4 cups of boiling water.
Let it steep for 30 minutes, strain, drink 2 cups a day.

Mix the following ingredients
    1 tsp. vitex berries.
    1 tsp. wild yam rhizome.
    ½ tsp. burdock root.
    ½ tsp. dandelion root.
    4 cups of boiling water.
Steep for 30 minutes, strain and drink 1 or 2 cups a day.

* Jamaican dogwood is a strong pain reliever, sedative and anti-spasmodic. Very helpful for muscular back pain, asthma, menstrual pain, insomnia, toothaches and nervous conditions.

Relaxing PMS Remedy.
1 tsp. Valerian rhizome tincture.
½ tsp. catnip leaves tincture.
½ tsp. passionflower leaves tincture.
1/4 tsp. peppermint leaves tincture.
Mix all ingredients and take a dropperful 4 times a day.

Menstrual cramp oil.

2 ounces Saint John's Wart oil.
8 drops Lavander essential oil.
8 drops Marjoram essential oil.
8 drops Chamomile essential oil.
Mix all ingredients and rub the lower obdomen with it as needed. This
formula can be used for back pain or any muscle related cramp.

Menstrual bleeding control tincture.

1 tsp. shepherd's purse leaf tincture.
1 tsp. yarrow leaf tincture.
1/2 tsp. red raspberry leaf tincture.
1/2 tsp. vitex berry tincture.
Mix all ingredients and take 1/2 a dropperful 4 times a day.

Stretch Marks:

It is very common that almost every woman at a specific time in her
life will develop stretch marks. Others simply have a generic
predisposition to stretch marks and get them everywhere while still
others never develop stretch marks at all.

They look like reddish lines across the body, and with time, they will
turn white. In pregnancy it is common to have them due to the fact
that the skin is stretching very rapidly to accommodate the baby and
the milk stored in the breasts.

Once the stretch marks develop they will stay with you forever; however, with time they will be less noticeable. The only way to avoid stretch marks is to prevent them.

We recommend:

* It is very important to exercise in order to get rid of stretch marks; toning your muscles helps your skin firm thus preventing stretch marks.

* Make sure that in your diet you are getting plenty of protein and foods rich in Vitamin C and Vitamin E which promote good tissue growth.

* Massaging your body with olive oil or Vitamin E may help.

* You can also try this homemade recipe: Mix one ounce of carrier oil (try avocado, sweet almond, jojoba, they are the best) with seven drops of lavender and five drops of chamomile. Massage into the body.

* Apply cocoa butter and/ or elastin cream thoughout the body as directed on the label. These are very good for stretch marks.

Here is another good recipe:
½ cup virgin olive oil.
1/4 cup aloe vera gel.
liquid from 6 capsules of Vitamin E.
liquid from 4 capsules of Vitamin A.
Mix all the ingredients together in a blender. Then pour the mixture into a jar and store it in the fridge. Apply the oil externally all over the placcs where the stretch marks commonly appear (abdomen, hips, thighs and breasts). If you do this consistently every day, you may prevent stretch marks.

Varicose Veins:

Varicose veins are abnormally enlarged veins that appear close to the skin's surface. They occur usually in the calves and thighs and are the result of malfunctioning valves inside the veins often caused by prolonged pressure or obstruction of the veins.

Varicose veins can develop in people from standing or sitting for long periods of time, poor exercise, pregnancy, excessive weight, prolonged constipation, and habitually sitting with legs crossed. Also, heavy lifting puts increased pressure on legs increasing the likelihood of developing varicose veins. Heart failure, liver disease and abdominal tumors can contribute to the formation of varicose veins. Heredity is also a factor for many individuals. A deficiency of Vitamin C and bioflavonoids can weaken the collagen structure in the vein walls which can lead to varicose veins.

Varicose veins are very common and affect approximately 10% of the population. More women than men are affected. In some cases if varicose veins are not treated properly, some complications can emerge. The most common characteristics are: swelling, restlessness, leg sores, itching, leg cramps, feeling of heaviness in the legs and fatigue.

We recommend:

* Eat a balanced diet that includes plenty of fish, fresh fruits and vegetables. The diet also has to be low in fat and carbohydrates.

* Eat as many blackberries and cherries as you can. They help prevent varicose veins and if you have them they may ease the symptoms.

* Including ginger, onions, garlic and pineapple in your diet is beneficial.

* Your diet has to be high in fiber to prevent constipation and keep the bowels clean.

* Avoid as much as possible sugar, ice cream, fried foods, peanuts, junk foods, cheeses, tobacco, salt, alcohol, animal protein, and processed and refined foods.

* Do a daily routine of exercise. Walking, swimming and bicycling all promote good circulation. It is very important to maintain a healthy weight.

* Do not wear tight clothes because they restrict blood flow.

* At least once a day, elevate your legs above the heart level for 20 minutes to alleviate symptoms.

* Avoid standing or sitting for long periods of time, crossing your legs, doing heavy lifting and putting any unnecessary pressure on your legs.

* If you sit at a desk all day, make sure you take breaks to walk around. You can also flex your muscles and wiggle your toes to increase blood flow. If it is possible, try to rest your feet on an object that is elevated from the floor when seated.

* If you have to stand for long periods of time, shift your weight between your feet, stand on your toes, or take breaks and walk around to alleviate pressure.

* Elevate your feet, as much as possible, at home while watching TV or sitting down to read.

* To ease pain and stimulate circulation, fill a tub with cold water and simulate walking.

* Avoid scratching the itchy skin above varicose veins. This can cause ulceration and bleeding.

* After bathing, apply Castor oil over the varicose veins affected and massage into your legs from the feet up.

* Also herbs can play a key role in treating varicose veins. Here are some helpful herbs:

* Aloe vera gel is a cooling and soothing treatment for varicose veins.

* Bilberry supports the health of connective tissue.

* Bromelain can help reduce the risk of clot formation in the blood vessels.

* To improve the circulation in the legs, Butchers broom, ginkgo biloba, gotu kola and hawthorn berries are very good.

* To relieve pain and inflammation use Cayenne. It also expands blood vessels, reducing stress on the capillaries.

* To alleviate tissue swelling use Dandelion. Dandelion reduces water retention.

* To stimulate blood flow, bathe the affected areas in white oak bark herb tea 3 times daily or simmer, but do not boil, a strong tea and use it to make compresses. Apply to the painful areas.

Here are some home recipes that might help:
2 tsp black cohosh root.
4 tsp Ginkgo biloba leaves.
2 cups boiling water.
Combine the herbs. Pour the boiling water over the herb mixture; soak for 30 minutes, strain. Take 2 to 3 tbsp at a time, repeat up to 6 times daily to improve circulation.

Topical formula.

1 tsp ocotilo bark.
1 tsp yarrow.
1 tsp witch hazel bark.
2 cups of water.
Combine all ingredients in a pan and cover, boil until reduced to one cup; cool and strain. Apply topically to reduce discomfort. Use as needed.

Vein Reducer.

½ tsp horse chestnut powder.
2 cups water.
Mix and moisten a sterile cotton gauze cloth with the mixture. Rub gently over the affected area. This is to reduce discomfort over inflamed veins.

Wrinkles form when the skin thins and loses its elasticity. The appearance of some wrinkles is due to aging and is the most common skin problem for women. One of the first signs of wrinkles normally appear around the eye and is called " crow's feet." As time goes by the cheeks and lips are the next thing we notice. As we age, our skin becomes thinner and dryer, both factors contribute to the formation of wrinkles.

There are many factors that can contribute in the development of wrinkles some of which are: diet and nutrition, muscle tone, pollution, habitual facial expressions, chemicals, stress, improper skin care, and lifestyle habits such as smoking.

The most important factor is sun exposure which is your skin's worst enemy because it dries the skin and leads to the generation of free radicals that can damage skin cells. Research shows that 90% of what we think are signs of age are actually signs of over exposure to sunlight. Furthermore, approximately 70% of sun damage comes from everyday activities such as driving and walking to and from your car.

The ultraviolet-A rays that cause this enormous damage are present all day long in all seasons. These ultraviolet-A rays wear away the elasticity of the skin, causing wrinkling. The worst part is that the effects of the sun are cumulative, although they may not be noticeable for many years.

TIP: Did you know that natural beauty products are not always as advertised?

Manufacturers say that their products contain natural ingredients but the reality is that they contain tiny amounts compared to the artificial substances used. You find out by looking at the label of the product. The ingredients are listed in descending order, starting with the greatest amount contained. For example, a product may be labeled as rosemary, but the label shows only chemicals and artificial substances and not a drop of pure rosemary.

We recommend:

* Eat a balanced diet including fruits, vegetables, whole grain foods, seeds, nuts and legumes.

* Drink plenty of fluids every day. This help to keep the skin hydrated and flush away toxins.

* Obtain fatty acids from cold pressed vegetable oils.

* Avoid alcohol, caffeine and cigarettes. They dry the skin and encourage the development of wrinkles. Also the smoking habit uses the lips' muscles hundreds of times a day which contributes to wrinkling.

* Always protect your skin from the sun by applying a sunscreen with a sun protection factor (SPF) of at least 15 to all exposed areas of the skin.

* Avoid alcohol-based products. Use hazel or an herbal, floral water instead.

* Avoid using harsh soaps or solid cleansing creams. Use natural oils such as avocado oil to remove dirt and makeup.

* Do not apply heavy oils around the eye area before going to bed. Because it might cause the eye to be puffy in the morning.

* Take Vitamin E to protect against free radicals that can damage the skin and contribute to aging and wrinkles.

* Take Vitamin C to promote the formation of collagen, a protein that gives the skin flexibility. It also fights free radicals and strengthens the capillaries that feed the skin.

* Take Silica. It is important for skin strength and elasticity and also, stimulates collagen formation.

* Take Vitamin A. It is necessary for healing and the construction of new skin tissue.

* Take Vitamin B complex + Vitamin B12. They are anti stress and anti aging vitamins.

* Take primrose or black currant seed oil. They are good healers for dermatitis, acne and others skin disorders.

* Use a collagen cream because it is very good for dry skin.

* Use elastin cream to help smooth existing wrinkles and prevent the appearance of new ones.

* To alleviate puffy eyes, peel a cucumber, cool it and place it in the eye area for 10 minutes. Repeat if necessary.

* To cleanse the pores, rub mush tomatoes over your face, then rinse.

* To protect your skin from free radical damage, add a few drops of green tea extract to your lotions or astringents.

* To moisture your skin, mash together grapes and honey, enough to make a paste, apply over your face as a mask. Leave it for 30 minutes then rinse away.

* To remove dead cells and improve skin texture, rub a small handful of dry short grain rice against your face for a couple of minutes.

* To soften and nourish the skin, mash half an avocado and apply over the face. Leave it on until it dries, then rinse with warm water.

Pregnancy the most special time for you, your partner and your baby, who in just 40 weeks will be coming into your life for ever. This is a time to be treated with great respect and awe. This is a time to do the best for you and your baby.

For your baby, this time of peace and security will depend upon our lifestyle and the lifestyles of those around you.

Tip: Studies have shown that women who are more fit tend to have shorter, easier labor.

What you eat and drink will construct your baby's body. Also mother nature ensures that it will do the very best that can be done in the physical developments of you and your child but much of the responsibility lies on the parent's shoulders. Special care can and should be taken and herbs can play a key role in this important time of your life.

Nature offers an abundance of plants and herbs for all the stages of your birthing process. Some plants or herbs may be used at specific times and others throughout your pregnancy, to ease, aid and tone the tissue and to facilitate the birth itself.

We all know that synthetic drugs are to be avoided during pregnancy. That's why a natural approach to healing should be considered throughout the time the baby's in the mother's womb. Natural techniques can help you increase your energy, consolidate emotional serenity and also help you deal with the comforts and problems that may emerge as you proceed through your pregnancy and prepare for the birth of your baby. This involves a good diet, regular exercise and plenty of rest.

During your pregnancy is the right time to consider the practice of other techniques such as massage sessions, herbalism, homeopathy, acupressure, visualization, and other mind/body techniques that can make your pregnancy easier and more comfortable for you and for your baby as well.

In this part of the book we'll offer precise amounts of herbs, homeopathic remedies and aroma therapy oils that will help you find a cure for some problem that might emerge or to just relax during this beautiful experience, as well as suggested dietary or vitamin/mineral supplementation.

Back Pain:

About 80% of adults suffer from back pain at some time in their lives. Backaches are categorized as acute and chronic. Acute pain is caused by movement or excessive use of the back which can injure the muscles, ligaments, bones, tendons.
Chronic pain is a recurring backache that restricts of normal movements for no particular reason and can also affect the tendons, ligaments and bones.

Problems with some organs can cause back pain as well, for example, kidney infection, prostate problems, female pelvic disorder, bladder and even constipation can be felt in the lower back.

Back pain is very common during pregnancy due to the considerable anatomical changes and stress in the body. Carrying a child changes the position of your internal organs putting a huge amount of pressure on the lower spine. The increase in body weight, the muscle relaxing effects of the hormone progesterone and the change in your center of gravity contribute to the problem. That's why every day as your baby grows it's harder to get up and down from chairs and beds.

If you have back pain you can also feel muscle aches, locked areas in your back, stiff neck and your whole body will ache.

Other causes of back pain can be poor postural habits, strains, microtrauma, muscle tension and nutritional deficiencies. When repeated episodes of injury are added to this mix, the discs become thin, deteriorated or ruptured. These events can also lead to arthritic related conditions. With nerves close by, swelling or compression in the spine often results in neuritis, lumbar neuralgia, or sciatica.

Herbal medicines are used in these conditions with far more safety then drugs especially in pregnant women.

We recommend

*Ask someone to massage the affected area with herbal oils using knuckles and increasing pressure slowly. After a few minutes you will feel less discomfort. This gets rid of tension and relaxes the muscles in that area.

*Every time you lift something, remember to bend your knees first. This will prevent your lower back from getting tense and causing damage to your spine and back muscles.

*Never twist while lifting as this can have a bad effect on your vertebrates.

*Avoid lifting heavy objects in the last couple of weeks of your pregnancy.

*Do not sit in couches. Always sit in firm chairs supporting the lumbar area with a pillow. This will help you keep your waist and lower back in the proper position.

*Apply St. john's Wort directly to the back area. CAUTION: Do not suntan as this oil makes your skin very sensitive to the sun.

*Do not wear high heel shoes. They change your center of gravity even more, increasing the risk of falling and they put more pressure on your back. Instead wear well fitted, well-padded flat shoes that support your feet and provide ample room for your toes.

*Try to sleep with pillows supporting your back, legs and belly.

*Here are some homeopathic remedies that will help you with back pains, Cimicifuga, Kali carbonica. Lincopodium, Nux vomica and Arnica.

*Black Haw contains compounds very similar to the ones found in aspirin. It relieves spasms and neuralgia of back and neck, sciatica, leg cramps, tension headaches and wry neck.

*Boswellia is a strong anti-inflammatory which reduces stiffness and pain. It has to be used for at least 4 weeks in chronic cases. It improves circulation around ligaments, joints and tendons.

*Jamaican dogwood is a strong pain reliever, sedative and antispasmodic. It's very helpful for muscular back pain, asthma, menstrual pain, insomnia, toothaches, and nervous conditions.

*Dong quai has 1.5 times the analgesic activity of aspirin. It relieves back pain, cramping, muscular spasms and inflammation.

*The herb Cat's claw grows in South America has been researched and proven to reduce inflammation while boosting the immune system. The studies also discovered that cat's claw contains anti arthritic compounds and is currently being used to treat people with rheumatoid arthritis.

*Take Vitamin E to protect and improve joint mobility.

*Bromelain comes from the stem of the pineapple. It contains anti-inflammatory blocks, reduces swelling, pain and damage to joints. A study done on 200 people showed a 75% greater reduction in inflammation than the ones obtained using drugs. Finally in the last few years bromelain is being used in hospitals across U.S.

*Wild yam, is used for back pain characterized by sharp, knifelike sensations.

*Barberry is used for low back pain often related to kidney weakness. Good also for sciatica and neuralgia with radiating pain.

*Horsetail has high amounts of silica which is essential for bones and connective tissue.

*Eat alfalfa or take alfalfa extract in capsules. It contains all the necessary nutrients to alleviate back pain.

TIP: A home made ice pack can be made by mixing 2 parts water and 1 part alcohol in a nylon bag and freezing it. The bag will be flexible thus molding to the body and it will not sweat.

*When pain hits suddenly, drink two large glasses of pure water. Dehydration can cause back pain.

*Several studies done in Scandinavia on smoking and non smoking twins have shown that smoking greatly aggravates problems in the disks. It's always advisable to quit smoking.

*Rhus toxicodendrom is a homeopathic remedy that relieves stiffness.

Breast-feeding:

Breast-feeding is the act of naturally feeding an infant with milk produced in the mother's breast. This has great deal of benefits for the baby. Not only is breast milk healthier but the action of feeding the child is a moment of love in which the baby learns to bond, smell, and caress with his or her mother as she gives nourishment and affection.

Without a doubt breast milk is the best food for a newborn, nothing comes closer to providing all the nutrients that the baby will need later in life. Breast milk is much easier to digest then any formula on the market, and at the same time it provides protection against infections, prevents future food allergies, helps the growth of healthy teeth, and most important it improves brain development. Studies have shown that breast-fed babies are more intelligent than formula fed babies.

However, many mothers stop breast-feeding after the third or fourth month switching to formula and later to cows' milk. This certainly robs the baby of the special qualities that breast milk offers. Infants that stop nursing before the forth month are at risk of developing asthma, food and respiratory allergies, intestinal bacteria, and oral weaknesses (poor tooth development).

Sometimes a mother cannot breast-fed her baby due to a number of reasons, such as, low quality of milk, breast pain, infection, etc. That's when herbs come into play, many midwives have used them for years to improve quality and quantity of milk, to fight infection and much more. Take a look at the following conditions and the natural ways to treat them.

Low quality or quantity of milk

Low quality of milk can be caused by medications or a poor diet. Many antibiotics contaminate the milk and a diet high in caffeine may cause colic and sleeping problems. For the baby, it's very important that the mother keeps eating a well balance diet after giving birth, and preferably foods with no traces of pesticides. These poisons become highly concentrated in the milk.

The use of a breast pump may inhibit the production of milk, lowering the amount available to the baby, this gives the false idea that the infant should be changed to formula in order for it to be satisfied when, in fact, the problem is the quantity of milk that the mother is producing.

Herbs can help with both of these common problems.

We recommend

* Eat alfalfa or take it in capsules, it stimulates lactation, improves quality and quantity of milk.

* Chaste tree increases flow of milk by affecting pituitary's prolactin secretion.

* Chinese use a herb called codonopsis to increase lactation and strengthen the blood.

* Goat's rue is an herb that has been used by midwives for hundreds of years to improve breast milk production by as much as 50%.

* Vervain encourages milk secretion and flow. It also increases absorption of nutrients from food and helps with postpartum depression.

* Milk thistle promotes production of milk and decreases pesticide residues in breast and milk.

TIP: Did you know that tight bras may stop the milk production and cause plugged ducts?

* Cumin helps increase milk production.

* Caraway, aniseed, dill, and fennel promote flow of best milk. It can be taken in form of teas or infusion.

* If you are prone to chills while breast-feeding and have poor quality of milk, use calcarea.

Milk Production Tea.

1 tsp. vitex berries.
1 tsp. blessed thistle leaves.
1/2 tsp. nettle leaves.
1/4 tsp. fenugreek seed.
1/4 tsp. anise seed.
1 quart boiling water.
Mix all ingredients and steep for 20 minutes. Strain and drink 2 cups a day.

Engorgement

Breast engorgement is a very common problem that starts affecting the mother in the first two or three weeks after delivery and is more annoying to women with poor skin elasticity. Engorgement is due to milk excessively filling the breast together with blood and fluid retention in the same area.

Usually the breast feels full, hard, tight, tender, painful, the breast feels hot to the touch and a fever may develop. The baby may also have a hard time to latch on and suck.

We recommend

* Take a handful of Confrey leaves and steam them for a few minutes wrapped in a gauze. Place on the breast for help in relieving engorgement.

* Take the homeopathic remedy Belladonna 6X.

* Soak a towel in hot water and place it on the breast ten minutes before feeding.

* Poke roots reduce swollen breast and pain. Use under doctor supervision.

* Elder is used to reduce swelling of engorged breast.

* Chamomile helps control inflamed breast.

* Give your baby frequent feeds on both breasts, 10 to 15 minutes each.

* Use a pump to extract milk between feedings to control engorgement.

* Massage the breast while feeding to help milk flow easily.

Mix 2 quarts of boiling water.

2 tsp. of vitex berries.
2 tsp. of blessed thistle leaves.
1 tsp. of nettle leaves.
½ tsp. fenugreek seed.
½ tsp. anise seed.
Let it steep for 30 minutes, strain and drink 2 cups a day.

* Bryonia reduces swollen and hard breasts.

* Pulsatilla and calcarea are very helpful reducing the size and hardness of engorged breasts.

* When the production of milk is excessive and produces engorgement, a cold compress using peppermint oil should be used.

* A compress of marshmallow and slippery elm often reduces engorgement.

Plugged Ducts

This is a problem that occurs when the baby does not empty the breast completely on each feeding. The milk remaining in the duct hardens and blocks the duct eventually plugging it. Tight bras can cause plugged ducts as well. If the breast feels sore, it might be a sign of plugged ducts. A plugged duct should be taken care of as soon as possible, otherwise it can develop into Mastitis.

We recommend

* Castor oil helps with inflammation and pain.

* Elder is used to reduce swelling of plugged breast ducts.

* Queen's Delight clears congestion of lymphatic vessels and, stimulates white blood cells to react to infection.

* Check your nipples every day. If you see dry milk on them or dark dots remove them with a cotton ball and warm water and feed your child as soon as possible from that breast.

* Place the baby in different positions every time. This will ensure that all ducts are being used.

* Place hot towels on the breast or run hot water over them in the shower.

* Massage the breast in the direction of the nipple to try to get the milk to come out.

Mastitis

Mastitis is a condition that results when a plugged duct becomes infected. The breast swells due to some bacteria that enters through tiny cracks on the nipples. The breast infected with mastitis becomes red and painful with pus secretion. Other symptoms are fever, fatigue, vomiting or nausea.

We recommend

* Take poke roots this helps mastitis. Use under doctor supervision.

* Queen's Delight clears congestion of lymphatic vessels, stimulates white blood cells to react to infection.

* Place hot towels on the breast or run hot water over them in the shower.

* Elder is used to reduce swelling of breast infected with mastitis.

* Rest as much as you can.

* Drink lots of water or alfalfa juice.

* Coat your nipples with breast milk after feeding.

* There are antibiotics that are safe for nursing mothers and their babies. See your doctor if your case is very severe. However, we recommend that you try to avoid antibiotics as much as you can.

* Wash your hands before and after feeding to prevent bacterial contamination.

* Dandelion is very helpful and a popular herb to treat mastitis.

* The Chinese use gentian to cure mastitis.

* Madder root is useful in relieving mastitis.

Cracked Nipples

Cracked nipples can develop when the baby is being positioned wrongly or by using damp breast pads. The nipple becomes irritated, red, and painful and in some cases, bleeding may develop.

* Calendula cream will soothe and encourage the healing of cracked nipples and is safe for the baby to swallow.

* The homeopathic remedy called chamomilla helps heal cracked nipples.

* The homeopathic remedy called pulsatilla helps heal cracked nipples.

* Sulfur is also helpful for cracked nipples.

* Apply vitamin E to sore and cracked nipples.

Morning Sickness:

Approximately 50% of all pregnant women experience nausea and vomiting between the sixth and the twelfth week of pregnancy. It's completely normal and can occur at any time of the day although it is called morning sickness. But one in 300 women will have severe abnormal vomiting which is continual nausea and vomiting after the twelfth week. This type of vomiting is called Hiperemesis gravidarum and it can result in dehydration, acidosis, malnutrition and weight loss. This condition can be dangerous to the fetus if it persists. The reason for Hiperemesis gravidarum has not been identified yet but an association between high levels of the hormones estrogen and chronic gonadotropin (HCG) has been found. HCG is a hormone produced by the placenta that increases until the end of the first trimester.

Other possible problems related with abnormal to severe vomiting includes bile duct disease, drug toxicity, pancreatitis, low blood sugar, problems with the thyroid and inflammatory bowel disorders.
In a more natural term, morning sickness is seen as a cleansing of toxins from the system that is preparing for pregnancy.

We recommend :

* Eat frequently during the day (at least six small meals daily) to help you avoid an empty stomach.

* Low blood sugar aggravates the nausea so you should try to keep a good level throughout the day staring from the moment you wake up. You can keep some crackers on your night table and eat them before you get up.

* Instead of eating your foods, try to drink them, it's easier for your body to digest a milk shake or fruit shake instead of having to chew them.

* Avoid foods and odors that make you feel nausea.

* Drink plenty of carbonated beverages without caffeine. Consuming ginger ale for example will promote the elimination of gas. Ginger ale contains ginger, a herb that soothes the digestive tract.

* Also mix single drops of ginger, fennel and peppermint oils, then add them in an ounce of carrier oil. This exquisite oil massaged into the skin will settle the stomach.

* For something more relaxing, put a few drops of lavender oil in the bath tub and enjoy the immersion.

* Taking ½ to 1 tsp of Wild yam root every day will help you deal with your morning sickness.

* A good tea can be made mixing equals parts of two or three of these herbs: Fennel, Cinnamon, Peppermint or Raspberry.

* Another useful tea can be made mixing :
   2 tsp Meadowsweet
   1 tsp Black Horehound
   1 tsp Chamomile
Take a china or glass teapot which has been previously warmed, add one teaspoonful of the dried herb mixture into it for each cup of tea that you intent to brew. After that, pour a cup of boiling water in for each teaspoonful of herb that is already in the pot and then put the lid on. Let it settle for 10 minutes approximately.

* Important*:Infusions may be drunk hot because that is the best way of obtaining results from a medicinal herbal tea. But they can be drunk cold or you can have ice in them if desire. They may be sweetened with honey, brown sugar or Licorice Root.

* During your pregnancy it's important to take the correct vitamins and minerals that will help you and your baby to be healthy. Here are the required during your pregnancy:

Vitamin A: 5,000 IU   Vitamin K: 65 mg
Vitamin B1: 1.5 mg   Folic Acid: 800 mcg
Vitamin B2: 1.6 mg   Calcium: 1,200 mg
Vitamin B3: 17 mg   Magnesium: 500 mg
Vitamin B6: 2.2 mg   Iron: 30 mg
Vitamin B12: 2.2 mcg   Phosphorus: 1,200 mg
Vitamin C: 500-1,000 mg   Iodine: 175 mcg
Vitamin D: 400 IU   Selenium: 65 mcg
Vitamin E: 400 IU

In addition take the following vitamins in complement with these:

* Vitamin B6 (25 mg) with Vitamin C (250 mg) and Vitamin K (5 mg) twice daily to prevent morning sickness.

* There is another supplement that you can take to prevent morning sickness which is L-Methionine and the suggested dosage is 1,000 mg daily.

* Next we'll describe some homeopathic remedies:

* If you find yourself vomiting with anxiety and you feel it right into your stomach, or if you can't stand the smell of food because it makes you nausea, you are always very thirsty or in the moment after eating or drinking cold beverages you feel worse, take Arsenicum.

* If right after eating you have sudden spasmodic vomiting and if you see mucous in your vomit, take Antimonium Tartaricum.

* If every time you have nausea or vomits you burp, if you have cravings for sweets and if you feel better outdoors, take Argentrum Nitricum.

* If you don't tolerate the smell or thought of food although you want or feel the necessity of eating them, or you have severe nausea from the sight of food, you feel thirsty and if your condition gets worse every time you move, take Colch.

* If you have the desire to vomit but can't, or your vomit is violent if you are constipated, irritable, or every time you eat your condition gets worse take, Nux Vomica.

* If you vomit but still have good appetite or feel uninterested and fatigued take Sepia.

* If you have nausea, chills and profuse salivation, take Tabacum.

Common Ailments

In this section we will tell you how to treat the most common ailments that affect us all. It is important to know that you don't have to run to the pharmacy every time something hurts or someone gets sick. Most of the illness that we encounter on a daily basis can be treated without expensive synthetic drugs.

We all have seen the commercials in which a big laboratory tells us how wonderful their medicine is but right before the commercial is over, the actor lets us know about all the side effects caused by this wonder drug; things like constipation, dry mouth, vomiting, dizziness, diarrhea etc.

Perhaps you have heard about a pill that claims to grow hair in a very small number of people. This drug also causes some undesirable sex malfunctions. Or perhaps you know how a laxative works by irritating the walls of the colon thus giving you the runs.

If you do not agree with the theory that you need to cause a small harm to feel good, you will find this section very useful.

All the ailments listed here are treated with natural herbs, vitamins, foods, and minerals. That's right, we use only mother nature's tools to cure ourselves the way it was intended from the beginning of time.

This does not mean that we are against modern medicine. We believe, that in the past few years this technique has advanced a great deal and many drugs and treatments are necessary to improve our lives. We are against the "business" that makes people believe that the body needs help from chemicals in the form of drugs for every little illness.

We are giving knowledge so that you can see your body like it is, the most perfect machine ever invented and capable of fixing itself if we give it the chance. Even when we treat our bodies badly by smoking, eating the wrong things, drinking alcohol etc., the body is always trying to repair what's broken, from a bone to a cold.

A good example would be the common cold. We start sneezing, our nose runs, we cough, we get a fever, all signs that the body is healing itself. Our sneeze is used by the body to expel some strange invader trying to get inside our respiratory system. Our nose creates mucus to trap particles so that when we blow our nose, the particles are ejected. Fever is the way the body elevates its temperature to kill

a harmful virus that has made it inside.
So we go out and buy some medicines to get rid of these symptoms and suppress our immune system. We take them and we feel a little better but it takes the body a lot longer to heal itself.

Do you see what these drugs do? They target the symptoms that are uncomfortable but that's what the body does to protect and heal itself. Synthetic drugs stop the natural way. Using natural remedies we can boost our immune system by giving our body the tools and power to heal faster.

Acne

Acne is an inflammatory disorder of the sebaceous (oil) glands located under the skin. When for some reason glandular activity increases, for example puberty, the glands secrete a lot more sebum then normal. If on its way to the surface, the sebum becomes trapped under the skin, the gland breaks, spilling sebum. This irritates the under layers of the skin and some pimples forms. This is how acne begins to affect several body parts, like the face, back, neck or chest.

Oil gets to the surface by traveling up the hair shaft. When the pores become clogged with excess oil and dead cells, the opening narrows; this shuts off oxygen to the pores and encourages bacterial growth, infection and inflammation. Blackheads arise when trapped oil darkens as it oxidizes (although many people mistakenly believe that this darkening of the pore is cause by dirt). When pores are repeatedly clogged, they enlarge and change the skin's texture.

Acne, although common among teenagers, can occur at any time in life and can be caused by allergies, high sugar or diets high in fat. In women Acne can be developed from the use of contraceptives which cause hormone changes. Some drugs such as cortisone or anti epileptics can cause acne as well. In severe cases, it scars and pits the skin.

TIP: Some doctors prescribe a contraceptive pill for girls suffering of acne. This pill contains a hormone called estrogen. The drug suppresses the hormonal actions and produces some dangerous side effects: nausea, vomiting, headaches, weight gain and liver malfunctions.

Acne has become the most treated skin condition in the past few years due to the mental anguish and the impact to the person's self esteem. People who have had acne for a long time report feelings of being unattractive and are very self-conscious about their skin problem. Acne can cause many psychological effects such as low self-esteem, confusion and frustration, anger, depression and social withdrawal.

People suffering from acne often seek help from a dermatologist who almost immediately prescribes antibiotics which can cause terrible side effects, for example, Clindamycin can cause colitis which in turn causes among others bloody stools and in some cases can be fatal. The only drug proven to work in 90% of cases is Isotretinoin, however, it can cause severe side effects, such as nose bleed, dry skin, headaches, joint and muscle pains and the most dangerous, birth defects.

DID YOU KNOW   that Tetracycline can permanently stain teeth of unborn children?

The skin is the largest organ in the body. It is in charge of several jobs. One of them is to get rid of some toxins and waste through sweating. If the liver and kidneys can't handle the amount of toxins, then the skin takes over and begins discharging the extra waste. This can have an effect on the skin's health and can cause acne and other disorders.

We recommend

* Colloidal silver is used as a natural antibiotic. Take orally and apply directly on the affected area.

* Take garlic capsules. They boost the immune system and kill the bacteria found in acne.

* To help the liver eliminate toxins from the blood, take Burdock root and dandelion which contain inulin. This helps kill bacteria thus improving the skin.

* Take the homeopathic remedies Kali bromatum, Sulphur, Antimonium tartaricum and Herpa sulphuris. These help prevent the formation of pimples or quickly bring them to a head.

* Use Lavender oil and apply directly on the acne area.

* Put Tea tree oil on the acne affected skin. This is a natural antibiotic. It will destroy a broad range of invading microorganisms as effectively as benzol peroxide but without side effects. It reduces redness, itchiness and stinging.

* Eat foods high in fiber. This will keep the colon clean.

* Eat Shellfish, soybeans, sunflower seeds and nuts. These are all rich in zinc which is an antibacterial.

* Do not drink alcohol, soft drinks or caffeine. Do not eat eggs, chocolate, fried food, or fats.

* Anything containing sugar can produce what is called "skin diabetes" which leads to acne.

* Drinking lots of water helps clean the body by carrying out waste.

* Do not use electric shavers. They can scar the skin affected by acne.

* Do not wear oil based makeup. Use water based natural makeup instead.

* Some medical journals in Germany show that the herb called vitex berry reduces hormone levels and controls their actions.

* Remember that stress can also cause acne especially in adults. Try to control or avoid stress. Many studies have shown a reduction of acne in people using relaxation techniques.

* Mix chamomile, licorice, elder flowers and red clover to unclog pores and refine, soften and heal the skin.

Pimple remover solution.

½ cup of boiling water.
2 tsp. Epson salts.
6 drops of lavender essential oil.
Mix water and salts, once the salt is dissolved. Add lavender and soak a cotton cloth and compress on affected area. If cloth cools, soak it again and repeat several times.

Acne Killer (intensive care).

1 tsp. of goldenseal root (powdered).
30 drops of tea tree oil essential oil.

Mix ingredients and form a paste. Apply directly on the acne affected skin and let it dry for 20 minutes. Rinse with lukewarm water.

* If pimples are red and bleeding use calendula. This antiseptic herb prevents scarring, speeds healing and it reduces inflammation.

* Yellow dock can be used as a compress to extract pus from pimples and quickly cure infection.

* Oregon grape is an excellent herb for chronic acne. It prevents pitting scars.

* Red clover is safe for children and very potent. It's used in traditional skin cancer formulas. It's very good for acne on the nose, forehead and scalp. It helps control oily skin.

Acne Healing Juices to be used during a fast.

Fasting helps eliminate toxins from the body especially from the liver and kidneys; this method of cleansing reduces the workload of these organs which in turn work more efficiently, cleaner blood means that fewer impurities are excreted though the skin, thus reducing acne. Try the juices below during fasting as a complementary treatment to the home remedies for acne.

Juices and smoothies

Apple, celery and cucumber juice

Ingredients:

8 apples

1/2 cucumber

6 sticks celery

Directions: Juice all the ingredients. Pour into glasses. Makes approximately 1 pint.

Carrot and mango juice

Ingredients:

8 medium size carrots, peeled or scrubbed

2 large ripe mangoes, peeled and stoned

Directions: Juice the carrots, followed by the mango. Pour into glasses. Makes approximately 1 pint.

Carrot, apple and ginger juice

Ingredients:

8 apples, washed and chopped but not peeled

4 carrots, peeled or scrubbed

1 inch ginger root, peeled

Directions: Juice the apples, then the carrots and finally the ginger. Pour into glasses. Makes approximately 1 pint.

Alzheimer's disease

Alzheimer's disease is a common type of dementia, or decline in intellectual function. Once thought rare, Alzheimer's disease is now known to affect more than 4.1 million people in the United States. It afflicts 10 percent of Americans over 65 years of age and as many as 50 percent of those over 85 years old. However, the disease does not affect only the elderly, but may strike when a person is in his or her forties. Most people over forty are using some type of alternative or home remedies to prevent the early development of Alzheimer's disease.

What is Alzheimer's disease?

This disorder was first identified in 1906 by a German neurologist named Alois Alzheimer. It is characterized by progressive mental deterioration to such a degree that it interferes with one's ability to function socially and at work. Memory and abstract thoughts process are affected. Alzheimer's disease is irreversible and progressive disorder that since 1906 very little progress has been made by conventional medicine to slow or prevent it. However, there are many home remedies for Alzheimer's disease that have shown remarkable results in preventing and in some cases restore mental deterioration.

I have very pour memory. Do I have Alzheimer's disease?

Many people worry that their forgetfulness is a sign of Alzheimer's disease. The fact is that most of us forget where we put our car keys or our glasses or someone's birthday but this is not a sign of Alzheimer's disease. A few good example of the difference between forgetfulness and Alzheimer's is the following: If you forget where you put your car keys that is forgetfulness, if you do not remember whether or not you have a car, that is Alzheimer's, or if you forget where you put your glasses that is forgetfulness, if you do not remember whether or not you use glasses that is Alzheimer's. Forgetfulness is also very frustrating and can also be improved by using some very powerful home remedies for memory loss.

What causes Alzheimer's disease?

The precise cause or causes of Alzheimer's are unknown, but research reveals a number of interesting clues. Many of them point to nutritional deficiencies. For example, people with Alzheimer's tend to have low levels of vitamin B12 and zinc in their bodies. The B vitamins are important in cognitive functioning, and well known that processed foods have been stripped from this nutrients. In addition the average sixty year old person is likely to be taking between 8 and 10 prescription and over-the-counter drugs, these potential drug reactions and pour diet often interfere or adversely affect mentally and physically since many medications deplete crucial vitamins and minerals.

Low levels of antioxidants vitamin A and E and carotenoids are also present in people suffering from Alzheimer's. These nutrients act as free radicals scavengers; damage caused by free radicals may expose the brain cells to increased oxidative damage.

How can I treat Alzheimer's naturally with home remedies?

* According to a report published in the October 22, 1977 edition of the Journal of the American Medical Association (JAMA), Ginkgo biloba extract can stabilize and in some cases improve the mental functioning and social behavior of people with Alzheimer's disease. Take 100 to 200 mg of ginkgo biloba extract 3 times a day.

* The Chinese herb Qian Ceng to (Huperzia serata) increases memory retention. This is the same herb that is the source of huperzine A, and it is also known as club moss. Pure and standardized extracts of this herb have been shown to increase clear-headedness, language ability and memory retention in a significantly high percentage of subjects with Alzheimer's disease. It is a potent blocker of acetylcholinesterase, an enzyme that regulates the activity of acetylcholine, which is an important chemical of the brain that maintains healthy learning and memory functions.

* Valerian root improves sleep patterns when taken as bedtime.

* Eat a well balanced diet of natural foods and follow the supplementation program mention above.

* Folate and Vitamin B12 prevent elevated levels of homocysteine, a chemical that increases the risk for Alzheimer's disease and heart disease. This vitamin may be important for preventing or delaying the symptoms of Alzheimer's disease. This vitamin is added to cereal products Foods containing folate include avocados, bananas, oranges, asparagus, green leafy vegetables, and dried beans. B12 is found only in animal products. (Oily fish are very high in B12 and also have other nerve-protective properties.). I recommend 400 mcg of folic acid to reduce homocysteine, although one study suggested 800 mcg (.8 mg) a day is necessary to reduce homocysteine levels.

* Avoid alcohol, cigarette smoke, processed foods, and metal pollutants like aluminum, and mercury.

TIP: Did you know that in a study published in the British Medical Journal, smoking doubles the chances of developing dementia and Alzheimer's?

* The herbs balm and sage are being researched for possible beneficial effects and brain chemistry. Balm appears to simulate the neurological receptors that bind acetylcholine. Sage contains compounds that are cholinesterase inhibitors.

* Vitamin E can slow the progression of Alzheimer's disease by as much as 25% according to a study in 1997.

* A study conducted by the research department at Oakwood college in Alabama sowed that liquid aged garlic extract (kyolic) may be useful in the improvement of Alzheimer's disease symptoms.

Anemia:

Anemia is a decrease in your blood cell count and/or a decreased hemoglobin content in the blood. Since red blood cells are the ones responsible for carrying oxygen to the cells via the hemoglobin, a lower amount would mean low oxygen in all your body's tissues and your baby would get less oxygen as well. Anemia can be caused by blood loss which means that not enough red cells are being produced or that too many red cells are being killed off. During pregnancy, the blood volume in your baby increases by about 40%.

Most women during their pregnancy become anemic because their bodies are not producing enough red cells and it is usually caused by a nutritional deficiency. Late in the second trimester, the hematocrit decreases but this does not make you anemic. Hematocrit is the percentage of red blood cell volume of the total blood volume.

Usually anemia is due to iron deficiency but also can be caused by not having enough Vitamin B12; B6; Folic acid, and/or copper in your system. During your pregnancy blood counts will be done that will help to determine what vitamins or nutrients you are lacking but in some cases more specific tests are needed. These might include blood work for Iron; Vitamin B12; Ferritin; Iron binding capacity and folic acid level. Just taking Iron is not always the answer. That's why it's important to find out the real cause of Anemia from blood test. Anemia has the following symptoms:

*You feel fatigued.

*You feel dizzy.

*You lack vitality.

*You are short of breath.

*Your skin looks white as well as your gums and around your eyes.

If you have Anemia at the time of delivery you will be at risk of losing excessive blood and going into shock. Your baby also may have low amounts of Iron stored for the first month of life.

TIP: There is another type of Anemia called "Pica." In this kind of Anemia you may have rare cravings, for example you will want to eat substances other than food, such as, coal, dirt, starch or hair. This kind of Anemia is usually the sign of a nutritional deficiency.

We recommend:

*It's very important to get the proper nutrients into the body. Eat a diet rich in cereals, rice, pastas, dairy products (milk, yogurt and cheese), vegetables and fruits, meat, poultry and fish and finally dry beans, eggs, and nuts. These foods have been proven to help boost the immune system.

*Make sure you are eating plenty of iron rich food such as, liver, green leafy vegetables, beets, dried fruits, bran flakes, oysters, brown rice, lentils and molasses, raisins, prunes; breads and pastas made of whole grain flour.

*Avoid drinking coffee, tea and ingesting antacids, because they decrease iron absorption.

*Try to cook in iron pots; it is proven that doing it can increase significantly the amount of iron in your foods.

*During your pregnancy it's important to take the correct vitamins that will help you and your baby be healthy. Here are the following required during this period:

Vitamin A: 5,000 IU
Vitamin E: 400 IU
Vitamin B1: 1.5 mg
Vitamin K: 65 mg
Vitamin B2: 1.6 mg
Calcium: 1,200 mg
Vitamin B3: 17 mg
Magnesium: 500 mg
Vitamin B6: 2.2 mg
Iron: 30 mg
Vitamin B12: 2.2 mcg
Phosphorous: 1,200 mg
Folic Acid: 800 mcg

Iodine: 175 mcg
Vitamin C: 500-1,000 mg
Selenium: 65 mcg
Vitamin D: 400 IU

*In addition take an organic form of Iron (amino acid chelate): 100 mg of elemental Iron daily (Iron aspararte, citrate or picolinate), not the poorly absorbed sulphate which may cause constipation and/or stomach ache.

*Vitamin C (500 mg) is recommended to be taken with iron for better absorption. Desiccated liver tablets may be helpful as well and a Folic acid supplement with Vitamin B6 and B12 should be used to prevent anemia.

*Also herbs can help your body maintain a good level of iron, such as:

½ to 1 tsp. of the tincture of Yellow dock root three times daily, or
½ to 1 tsp. of extract of Dandelion leaf and/or root or two capsules twice daily, or
Eat Dandelion greens in your salads.

Here are some homeopathic remedies:

*Take China if the cause of the anemia is due to loss of blood or fluids.

*If your skin looks pale or white, shiny or a little green, take Calcarea Phosphoric.

*If your face looks red and then suddenly turns pale and your feet and hands swell take Foram acet.

*To improve the quality of your red blood cells in your body take Foram Phosphoric which can also be taken with Calcarea Phosphorica.

*If you take Calcarea Phosphorica use a 3X potency that will help you build up your hemoglobin level.

*If your gums look white and your blood rushes to your head when you lay down take Graphite.

*If your body feels cold and chilly or if the cause of your anemia is due to loss of blood because you have menstrual disorders take Natrum Muriaticum.

*If you are not thirsty and your body is cold and you feel tired and your condition improves being outdoors take Pulsatilla.

*Eat alfalfa. This nutritive herb promotes digestion/assimilation of vitamins minerals. An excellent source of nutrients, it's needed for iron absorption and blood clotting including B6, E, K, Iron, potassium, zinc, magnesium.

*Dong Quai is a Chinese herb rich in B12 and folic acid. It treats iron deficiency anemia increases the production of red blood cells and combats weakness and fatigue. It also protects the liver.

*For anemia after or before childbirth use Raspberry leaf. it is very rich in iron and calcium and also helpful for excess loss of blood due to injury or menstruation.

*A very good blood tonic is found in the herb called yellow dock. It assists in the assimilation of dietary iron.

Arthritis

Arthritis is a prehistoric disease; archeologists have found skeletons of the first humans with evident cases of arthritis. But modern medicine has not yet found the reason why this condition affects more then 100 million people around the world.

Arthritis affects the joints of the body. They become swollen, painful, deformed and stiff and eventually the joint loses range of motion and the pain becomes unbearable. There are many types of arthritis; the most common one is Osteoarthritis which causes a slow deterioration of the cartilage on the tip of each bone. The bones then start rubbing against each other injuring the articulation and scar tissue grows to deform the area.

There are several drugs that deal with the pain and inflammation of arthritis but most of them don't do a very good job considering all the side effects they cause. For example ibuprofen (Advil) or naproxen (Aleve) and even other more powerful prescription drugs cause severe gastrointestinal problems such as bleeding ulcers, acidosis and stomach pain. They interfere with the synthesis of collagen which is fundamental for the formation of cartilage. If cartilage is not rebuilding itself more damage is going to be inflicted on the joints.

Although the commercials on television tell us it is safe to take over the counter drugs every day and many people suffering from arthritis do, the truth is that they cause damage to other parts of the body which is a price too high to pay just too high to temporarily get rid of pain and inflammation.

But not everybody knows this. When they start to experience gastrointestinal problems a drug is prescribed to deal with that condition suppressing the stomach acid in order to cure the ulcers in their stomach. This causes incomplete digestion (not enough acid to dissolve food) which leads to an insufficient absorption of nutrients, low level malnutrition, fatigue and depressed immune systems. At this point a person can be taking anywhere from 6 to 10 pills a day, then quality of life starts to go downhill just because they have arthritis pain.

Some people suffering all these side effects opt to take acetaminophen (Tylenol) because it works blocking the nerve impulses to the brain that trigger the pain sensation. This drug will not cause ulcers and gastrointestinal bleeding. The problem is that it does not control inflammation and an inflamed joint with no pain sensation is likely to be severely damaged because you don't feel the pain and you push the joint to perform resulting in grater damage to the whole articulation.

If you are one of the lucky ones who don´t have gastrointestinal problems you still need to be careful bacause these drugs also cause liver and kidney damage when used daily for prolonged periods of time.

There is a drug called celecoxib (Celebrex) this is one big money maker to the drug company, in the first three months in the market it was prescribed to about 2.5 million people in the United States alone. This is a very expensive drug about 2 US$ per pill and still has severe side effects. It's been linked to more then ten deaths, half of them due to gastrointestinal hemorrhage. The FDA has requested that the safety information of all of these products include information about cardiovascular and gastrointestinal risks.

Since there is no cure for arthritis and the risk of damage that could be generated by drugs is great, we suggest that you take a good look at all the natural remedies that have been with us since the year 500 AD. Mother earth gives us some very powerful herbs that can reduce arthritis pain and inflammation and combined with nutrients, mineral and vitamins are sure to get rid of the symptoms of arthritis without side effects and without chemicals.

We recommend

TIP: Any kind of infection anywhere in the body can contribute to causing Arthritis.

* Eat Alfalfa or take alfalfa capsules. It's very rich in minerals needed for the formation of bones.

* Take chondroitin sulfate 700 mg. a day to strengthen joints and ligaments.

* Take Vitamin E to protect and improve joint mobility.

* Bogbean is a very powerful aquatic herb for for rheumatoid arthritis and Osteoarthritis It is anti-inflammatory and cleans the urinary tract so drink lots of water.

* Boswellia has anti-inflammatory effects similar to Non-steroidal anti-inflammatory drugs (NSAID) (Advil, Aleve, Tylenol etc.) but this herb does not have side effects and does not cause gastrointestinal bleeding. It improves circulation to the joints, relieves pain, inflammation and stiffness.

* Ginger is the Killer of Arthritis pain. Superior to any NASID, it can be applied directly on the affected area or taken orally, either way it relieves pain, inflammation, stiffness, bursitis and tendinitis.

* Curcumin stimulates the production of cortisone better or equal to cortisone and anti-inflammatory drugs. It's an antioxidant and anti-inflammatory especially good for rheumatoid arthritis and Osteoarthritis. Take it orally or externally.

* Cayennes is very helpful for pain. Use it as an external ointment. It improves circulation.

* Bromelain comes from the stem of the pineapple and contains anti-inflammatory blocks, reduces swelling, pain and damage to joints. A study done on 200 people showed a 75% reduction in inflammation which is better than that obtained using drugs. In the last few years Bromelain has been used in hospitals across U.S.

Arthritis pain relief remedy.

Mix 2 tsp. of devil's claw tuber.
    2 tsp. of white willow bark.
    1 tsp. feverfew.
    2 tsp. yucca root.
    2 tsp. sarsaparilla root.
    3 cups of water.
Soak all ingredients in the water for eight hours, drain and drink 1/2 a cup 3 times a day.

* Du Huo Gashing is a Chinese herbal medicine that has proven to be helpful for arthritis.

* Nettle leaf is used in Germany for arthritis.

* A combination of ash bark, aspen bark and goldenrod has been used in Germany for 30 years to treat arthritis.

* Eating 20 cherries a day is more effective than Aspirin in relieving pain and inflammation.

TIP: Women with silicone breast implants are at a very high risk of developing antibodies that can attack collagen causing damage to joints, tendons and ligaments.

* To repair and rebuild bones and cartilage, eat foods rich in sulfur such as eggs, garlic and onion.

* Eat fresh pineapple. As mention before it contains Bromelain, an anti-inflammatory enzyme.

* Vitamin D3 is needed for good bone formation. Remember that the sun gives it for free. Spend time outdoors in order to get sunshine because it promotes the synthesis of vitamin D3.

* Soak a cotton rag in hot castor oil wrap the affected area with the cloth, place a piece of plastic over it and apply a heating pad to keep the oil warm. This is very helpful in relieving stiffness and pain.

* Combining the Chinese herbs blupleurum, ginseng and licorice will be very helpful in reducing or completely relieving pain resulting from inflammation. These herbs reverse the damage caused by the drug Prednisone which is used for the same condition but the herbs produce no side effects.

* The herb Cat's Claw grows in South America has been researched and proven to reduce inflammation while boosting the immune system. These studies also discovered that cat's claw contains anti-arthritic compounds and is currently being used to treat people with rheumatoid arthritis.

* Injections made with the herb Devil's claw are prescribed by physicians in Europe. It's also used in ointment and tea to reduce arthritis pain and inflammation.

Inflammation and pain Tincture.

1/2 tsp. of bupleurum root tincture.
1/2 tsp. of ginseng root tincture.
1/2 tsp. of licorice root tincture.

1/2 tsp. of echinacea root tincture.

1/2 tsp. of yucca root tincture.

Combine all ingredients and take half a dropperful three times a day.

Acute Bronchitis Home Remedies

The lungs are among the body's largest organs. The air we breathe enters our bodies through the trachea (windpipe), which connects with the bronchi, the breathing tubes that lead into the alveoli (air sacs) in the lungs. In the lungs, air is exchange for carbon dioxide.

Bronchitis is an inflammation or obstruction in the bronchial tubes. This inflammation results in a buildup of mucus, along with coughing, fever, pain in the chest area and / or back, fatigue, sore throat, difficulty breathing, and, often, sudden chills and shaking. Bronchospasm, a contraction of the smooth muscle in the walls of the bronchi, may also occur. Swelling of the mucous membranes and hypersecretion by the bronchial glands frequently accompany bronchospasm.

Bronchitis can be either acute or chronic. Acute bronchitis is usually cause by an infection, which can be bacterial, viral, chlamydial, mycoplasmal, or caused by combination of agents. It typically follows an upper respiratory tract infection, such as a cold or influenza. In acute bronchitis, bronchospasm is more often associated with viral (rather then bacterial) infection. Most cases of acute bronchitis are self-limiting, with full recovery in a matter of weeks. In some cases, however, the condition can lead to pneumonia. This is more likely to occur in those who also have chronic respiratory disease or other debilitating health problems.

Chronic bronchitis results from frequent irritation of the lungs, such as from exposure to cigarette smoke, air pollutants, or other noxious fumes, rather than from infection. Allergies may also be the cause of chronic bronchitis. Chronic bronchitis diminishes the exchange of oxygen and carbon dioxide in the lungs, so the heart works harder in an attempt to compensate. Over time, this can lead to pulmonary hypertension, enlargement of the heart, and ultimately heart failure.

Chronic bronchitis is one of the most common diseases seen by allergists, otolaryngologists, and primary care physicians. Specialists in an occupational medicine have long known that an adverse environment produces a vulnerability to respiratory infections. Climatic factors and epidemics of viral infections also increase the risk. Among people who live or work in unhealthy environments, shortness of breath is frequently aggravated by dampness and cold, exposure to dust, or even minor respiratory infections.

Most cases of pneumonia and bronchitis are not helped by antibiotics, since these drugs have no effect on viral infections. Medical researches have confirmed this fact in carefully controlled clinical studies. Nonetheless, 70 percent of doctors still give people antibiotics for acute bronchitis, based on misconceptions that doctors share with the general public. These include the common beliefs that a change in phlegm color from yellow to green is a sign of bacterial infection, or that antibiotics treatment for bronchitis will prevent the progress of the disease to pneumonia when actually both disorders can exist at the same time.

What nutrients are needed in order to recover from bronchitis faster?

As in most diseases natural therapies can help speed up the healing process of bronchitis, a conventional approach may be recommended as well, but without a doubt natural holistic medicine has a lot to offer to any bronchitis sufferer. Take in consideration al the nutrients we recommend below they are essential for a speedy recovery. They are organized in order of importance from essentials to important.

* Colloidal silver is a natural antibiotic that destroys bacteria, viruses, and fungi. It also promotes faster healing. Take as directed on the label, alternating one week on and one week off.

* Pycnogenol removes dangerous substances and protects the lungs. It is also a powerful antioxidant.

* Take Quercitin-C 500 mg 3 times a day. It is used for allergic bronchitis, it has an antihistaminic effect.

* Take vitamin A 20,000 IU twice a day for a month, then reduce the 15,000 IU a day. IMPORTANT: If you are pregnant do no exceed 10,000 IU a day.

* Natural Beta-carotene is needed for lung repair and protection. Take 50,000 IU a day.

* Vitamin C enhances immune function and reduces histamine levels. I recommend using it in buffered power form. Take 3,000 to 10,000 mg. a day in divided doses.

* Coenzyme Q10 improves circulation and breathing. Take 60 mg. a day.

* Clinical tests have shown that MSM (Mythylsulfonyl-methane) improves lung conditions such as bronchitis, pneumonia, emphysema, cysts or damage due to heavy smoking. Use as directed on the label.

* Vitamin E is a powerful oxygen carrier which improves breathing and repairs damaged tissue. Take 400 IU twice a day 50 – 100 mg. vitamin C.

* Garlic is a natural antibiotic that reduces infection and detoxifies the body. Take 2 tablets 3 times a day.

Herbal therapy to recover from bronchitis faster

Herbal medicine has proven to be very effective in the treatment of bronchitis. The following treatments may be very useful in alleviating some of the symptoms.

* American and Siberian ginseng are especially good for the lungs. They clear bronchial passages and reduce inflammation. Important: Do not use American ginseng if you have high blood pressure or any other heart problem.

* The plant horehound has been used for cough and lung congestion for many years; Horehound is largely used as expectorants and tonics. It is considered one of the most popular respiratory home remedy for bronchitis, being given with benefit for chronic cough, asthma and other respiratory problems.

Horehound is sometimes combined with hyssop, rue, liquorice root and marshmallow root, 1/2 oz. of each boiled in 2 pints of water, to 1 1/2 pint, strained and given in 1/2 teacupful doses, every two to three hours.

* Both American ginseng and Siberian ginseng clear the bronchial passages and reduce inflammation.

* Bromelain in tea form; it helps liquefy and decreases bronchial secretions; It also prevents the progression of bronchitis and sinusitis. Take 250 to 500 mg. 2 to 3 times a day between meals.

* Coltsfoot relieves acute congestions and hoarseness. Take only over the course of one week then discontinue. Make a tea in one cup of water and take 3 times a day.

* Lobelia breaks up bronchial congestion and stops wheezing. Take 500 – 1,000 mg capsules 3 times a day. Use only for two weeks and discontinue.

* Use essential 15 drops of lavender oil in a full bathtub, take and immersion bath for 20 minutes, it helps easy chronic bronchitis.

* Include plenty of onion and garlic to your diet, it has been shown that they contain quercetin and muster oils, which inhibit lipoxygenase, an enzyme that aids in releasing an inflammatory chemical in the body.

TIP: Did you know that dental plaque can serve as a reservoir for the bacteria that cause bronchitis? Regular dental cleaning can sharply reduce the incidence of bronchitis.

Instructions to do steam inhalation for bronchitis

* Pour hot water into a bowl and 3 drops of German chamomile and elderberry essential oil, place your head about 12 inches (30 cm) above the bowl and cover your head with a towel in such a way that the sides are totally closed and you in actual fact form a tent over the bowl.

Keep your eyes shut and breathe deeply through your nose for 1 to 2 minutes.

If you feel that the treatment is getting too much for you, raise the towel so that fresh air is brought into the area and breathe through your mouth a couple of times and then resume the treatment. If you at any time feel uncomfortable discontinue the treatment.

Basic recommendations

* Natural eucalyptus throat drops from the Swiss company Ricola help open the airways. I f you would rather use a homemade method you can inhale a few drops of eucalyptus essential oil 3 times.

* Do not swallow mucus; it should be disposed in a tissue. Swallowing mucus can bring stomach problems which in turn can depress the immune system even further.

* Do no use cough suppressants if you have bronchitis, coughing is a natural body function needed to excrete mucus secretions.

* Avoid smoking or secondhand smoke.

* A very common mistake by people suffering from bronchitis is that they don't wash their hands regularly. It custom and good manners to cover our mouth when we cough, not washing our hand helps spread the virus and delays the healing process.

TIP: Medication used to treat high blood pressure can cause life threatening complications in people with asthma.

Asthma is a very common respiratory disease. It affects the trachea and bronchial tubes which become inflamed and plugged with mucus. This causes the airways to narrow restricting the amount of air going to the lungs and makes it very difficult to breathe. Asthma can occur in anyone but is very common in children and early adulthood. Typical symptoms of an asthma attack are coughing, wheezing, tight chest and difficulty breathing.

There are two types of asthma: allergic and non allergic. Some of the allergens that can trigger an asthma attack are chemicals, drugs, smoke, dust, food additives, pollution, mold, etc. Non allergic asthma can be caused by anxiety, exercise, dry or humid weather, fear, laughing, stress etc.

The rate in which asthma attacks has increased in the past few years is alarming, especially in children. Scientists believe that there is a strong link between contamination in the air we breathe and asthma. Evidence suggests that the percentage of people who live in big cities and have asthma attacks is far greater than those of people who live in rural areas. However this may not be the only reason. Genetics food additives, toxins etc also play a part.

Modern medicine can offer very little to children with asthma. Most drugs can only produce a temporary effect. Herbs on the other hand can be very helpful not only reducing attacks but also strengthening the lungs and immune system. You'll learn to treat this disease with many combinations of herbs such as mullein, elecampane and more.

TIP: Did you know that aspirin, Advil, chemotherapy and antibiotics can cause asthma attacks?

We recommend

* Vitamin B6 and Vitamin B12. They are very important nutrients to treat asthma by decreasing the inflammation in the lungs.

* Vitamin C Is needed to fight infection, increase the amount of oxygen and reduce inflammation.

* Use ginkgo biloba. This herb contains ginkgolide B which is very helpful. Some studies indicate that ginkgo biloba reduces the frequency of asthma attacks.

* Mullein oil is used to fight respiratory congestion. It is very important to make it as a tea for faster results.

* Pau d'arco is a natural antibiotic and reduces inflammation.

* In China a powerful mixture of herbs called Shuan Huang Lian is being used in hospitals to treat respiratory illness. It is very important to use this herb to treat asthma and acute bronchitis.

* If exercise triggers asthma attacks, cut back the amount of salt in your diet and take 2,000 mg. of Vitamin C one hour before your workout.

* Eat salmon 3 times a week and take salmon oil capsules.

* Drink coffee and soft drinks with caffeine (colas). Caffeine dilates the bronchial airways.

Make a tea using:
2 tsp. powdered Indian root.
2 tsp. granulated echinacea root.
2 tsp. elecampane root.
2 cups of water.
Mix all ingredients and let them set for 2 hours.

To improve breathing

make a tea with:

1 quart boiling water.
1 tsp. chamomile flowers.
1 tsp. echinacea root.
1 tsp. mullein leaves.
1 tsp. passionflower leaves.
Mix herbs and pour boiling water over them, steep for 20 minutes, strain and give ½ a cup a day.

Throat spray for asthma attacks. (This remedy is used as many asthmatic inhalers).

1 tsp. ginkgo leaves (tincture form).
5 drops chamomile essential oil.
1/4 cup of water.
Mix all the liquids and store them in a spray or pump bottle to use as needed. This remedy keeps airways clear and dilated.

* A very tasteful herb for children is Lemon verbena tea. This herb reduces wheezing and doctors recommend it in South America.

* If you have a baby make sure you breast feed. This has been shown to greatly improve the chances of not getting asthma in the first place.

Chinese preparation remedy.

1 tsp. magnolia flowers.
1 tsp. rehmannia root.
½ tsp. don quai root.
3 cups of water.
Boil all ingredients and simmer for 15 minutes, remove from heat and steep for another 15 minutes, strain and give one cup a day.

* In recent studies scientists in Germany discovered that onion contains some compounds that are very helpful with asthma. Drink one glass of onion juice a day. If your child will not drink onion juice you can try to add onion to his or her food.

* Jamaican dogwood is a strong pain reliever, sedative and antispasmodic. It's very helpful for muscular back pain, asthma, menstrual pain, insomnia, toothaches, and nervous conditions.

Athlete's Foot:

TIP: Nursing mothers sometimes develop a fungus infection called Candida infection of the nipples. This causes severe pain while feeding and could be more complicated if the baby develops Oral Thrush, a fungal infection of the mouth which causes   mother and baby to reinfect each other.

Athlete's foot is a very common infection that affects mostly men and young people. It attacks the area between toes, soles of feet, fingernails and toenails. This infection is caused by a fungus called tinea pedis which lives off the dead skin cells and thrives in moist, warm places, such as gyms, locker rooms, showers and swimming pools. It is also very contagious and is transmitted by coming in contact with wet floors or by touching infected shoes or socks.

If repeated fungal infections are developed it might be a sign of fungus in the groin area. In these cases the problems should be treated simultaneously. Symptoms are: burning sensation between toes, itching, redness, scaling and blistering.

We recommend

* Add 40 drops of tea tree oil to a small amount of water and soak your feet in it for 10 minutes. Then dry the feet with a towel and a hair dryer to ensure that there is no moister present. This is important because the fungus might flourish under a toe nail that has not been completely dried. Place a few drops of oil on the area.

* Use olive leafs as an anti bacterial for infections.

* Take fresh garlic slices and put it in your shoes and wear it all day. This is the best way to cure athlete's foot, even better then all over the counter anti fungal drugs.

* Drink pau d'arco tea and soak your feet in a more concentrated form of about 10 tea bags.

* Do not wear socks twice without wasing them, and make sure to keep your feet dry.

Mix 2 tsp. of big sagebrush root.
    2 tsp. of white cedar leaf tips.
    1 cup of water.
Let it sit for 8 hours in a non metallic pot and apply to the area daily.

Antifungal vinegar.

4 ounces of oregano vinegar.
2 tbsp. of pau d'arco tincture.
1/4 tsp. tea tree oil essential oil.
1/4 tsp. lavender essential oil.
1/8 tsp. peppermint essential oil.
Mix ingredients and soak cotton balls in the liquid. Place on the affected area by athlete's foot.

Antifungal powder.

1/4 cup bentonite clay.
1/8 tsp. tea tree oil essential oil.
1/8 tsp. lavender essential oil.
Mix clay and oils in a plastic bag. Close the bag tightly and mix well by turning the bag over. Make sure to brake up clumps. Store for 2 days, then use as needed.

Back Pain:

About 80% of adults suffer from back pain at some time in their lives. Backaches are categorized as acute and chronic. Acute pain is caused by movement or excessive use of the back which can injure the muscles, ligaments, bones, tendons.
Chronic pain is a recurring backache that restricts of normal movements for no particular reason and can also affect the tendons, ligaments and bones.

Problems with some organs can cause back pain as well, for example, kidney infection, prostate problems, female pelvic disorder, bladder and even constipation can be felt in the lower back.

Back pain is very common during pregnancy due to the considerable anatomical changes and stress in the body. Carrying a child changes the position of your internal organs putting a huge amount of pressure on the lower spine. The increase in body weight, the muscle relaxing effects of the hormone progesterone and the change in your center of gravity contribute to the problem. That's why every day as your baby grows it's harder to get up and down from chairs and beds.

If you have back pain you can also feel muscle aches, locked areas in your back, stiff neck and your whole body will ache.

Other causes of back pain can be poor postural habits, strains, microtrauma, muscle tension and nutritional deficiencies. When repeated episodes of injury are added to this mix, the discs become thin, deteriorated or ruptured. These events can also lead to arthritic related conditions. With nerves close by, swelling or compression in the spine often results in neuritis, lumbar neuralgia, or sciatica.

Herbal medicines are used in these conditions with far more safety then drugs especially in pregnant women.

We recommend

*Ask someone to massage the affected area with herbal oils using knuckles and increasing pressure slowly. After a few minutes you will feel less discomfort. This gets rid of tension and relaxes the muscles in that area.

*Every time you lift something, remember to bend your knees first. This will prevent your lower back from getting tense and causing damage to your spine and back muscles.

*Never twist while lifting as this can have a bad effect on your vertebrates.

*Avoid lifting heavy objects in the last couple of weeks of your pregnancy.

*Do not sit in couches. Always sit in firm chairs supporting the lumbar area with a pillow. This will help you keep your waist and lower back in the proper position.

*Apply St. john's Wort directly to the back area. CAUTION: Do not suntan as this oil makes your skin very sensitive to the sun.

*Do not wear high heel shoes. They change your center of gravity even more, increasing the risk of falling and they put more pressure on your back. Instead wear well fitted, well-padded flat shoes that support your feet and provide ample room for your toes.

*Try to sleep with pillows supporting your back, legs and belly.

*Here are some homeopathic remedies that will help you with back pains, Cimicifuga, Kali carbonica. Lincopodium, Nux vomica and Arnica.

*Black Haw contains compounds very similar to the ones found in aspirin. It relieves spasms and neuralgia of back and neck, sciatica, leg cramps, tension headaches and wry neck.

*Boswellia is a strong anti-inflammatory which reduces stiffness and pain. It has to be used for at least 4 weeks in chronic cases. It improves circulation around ligaments, joints and tendons.

*Jamaican dogwood is a strong pain reliever, sedative and antispasmodic. It's very helpful for muscular back pain, asthma, menstrual pain, insomnia, toothaches, and nervous conditions.

*Dong quai has 1.5 times the analgesic activity of aspirin. It relieves back pain, cramping, muscular spasms and inflammation.

*The herb Cat's claw grows in South America has been researched and proven to reduce inflammation while boosting the immune system. The studies also discovered that cat's claw contains anti arthritic compounds and is currently being used to treat people with rheumatoid arthritis.

*Take Vitamin E to protect and improve joint mobility.

*Bromelain comes from the stem of the pineapple. It contains anti-inflammatory blocks, reduces swelling, pain and damage to joints. A study done on 200 people showed a 75% greater reduction in inflammation than the ones obtained using drugs. Finally in the last few years bromelain is being used in hospitals across U.S.

*Wild yam, is used for back pain characterized by sharp, knifelike sensations.

*Barberry is used for low back pain often related to kidney weakness. Good also for sciatica and neuralgia with radiating pain.

*Horsetail has high amounts of silica which is essential for bones and connective tissue.

*Eat alfalfa or take alfalfa extract in capsules. It contains all the necessary nutrients to alleviate back pain.

TIP: A home made ice pack can be made by mixing 2 parts water and 1 part alcohol in a nylon bag and freezing it. The bag will be flexible thus molding to the body and it will not sweat.

*When pain hits suddenly, drink two large glasses of pure water. Dehydration can cause back pain.

*Several studies done in Scandinavia on smoking and non smoking twins have shown that smoking greatly aggravates problems in the disks. It's always advisable to quit smoking.

*Rhus toxicodendrom is a homeopathic remedy that relieves stiffness.

High Cholesterol:

There are two types of cholesterol: Low density lipoproteins or LDL (bad cholesterol) and High density lipoproteins HDL (good cholesterol). LDLs are responsible for plaque buildup in the arteries which block the flow of blood to major organs like the liver, the kidneys, genitals and brain and is the number one cause of heart disease.

HDLs in the other hand are considered good because they carry unused cholesterol back to the liver where it was produced. Once there the liver breaks it down to be removed from the body. The needed cholesterol plays an important part in the formation of sex hormones and proper nerve and brain function. However if we do not have enough HDLs or too much cholesterol for them to pick up and transport back to the liver it will stay in our arteries blocking them.

But you are probably asking yourself if the cholesterol is produced in the liver, why would I have too much? It seems like the liver would regulate how much cholesterol is needed. That is right. The problem is that cholesterol is also present in our diet and usually we eat too much saturated fats such as coconuts, white bread, gravies, pork products, etc. and all these added to the cholesterol produced by the liver could make us reach an unsafe cholesterol level.

The number considered to be safe for both LDL and HDL is 200 mg./dl (milligrams per deciliter). A reading above 200 is a sign of potential development of heart disease, a level of 240 is considered to be at high risk. It is also important to maintain a good level of HDLs, 80 mg./dl. is recommended. A reading of 35 HDL would be considered very low even if the total level is below 200 mg./dl.

There are drugs to keep LDL levels low but these drugs can cause side effects including vomiting, headaches, Impotence, internal bleeding and vitamin deficiencies including Coenzyme Q10, the heart's most important nutrient. Why experience all that when there is a better way to keep cholesterol levels at an acceptable number. Taking herbs, vitamins and cutting fats from our diet is the safest way of ensuring a low risk of developing heart disease.

We recommend

Mix 1 tsp. of roasted chicory root.
      1 tsp. of lime flowers.
      ½ tsp. of fenugreek seeds.
      ½ tsp. of ginger rhizome.

1 quart of water.
Boil all ingredients, let cool, strain. Drink 2 cups a day.

* Eat Garlic or take 1 capsule twice a day. It lowers LDL cholesterol level by 12% and increases HDLs.

* Take 400 mcg. a day of chromium picolinate to improve HDL to LDL ratio.

* Taking 4000 mg. Vitamin C with bioflavonoids a day lowers cholesterol.

* Ginger reduces cholesterol and thins the blood improving circulation.

* Guggul reduces LDL by 35% and increases HDL by 20 % in 12 weeks to prevent arteriosclerosis. It has performed better then many drugs in several studies.

* Red Rice Yeast is a Chinese medicine that lowers cholesterol, improves circulation and strengthens the heart.

* Eat vegetables and fruits as they are cholesterol free.

* Spirulina taken daily has been shown to lower cholesterol.

* Olive oil, bananas, apples, carrots, dried beans, garlic and grapefruit are the cholesterol lowering foods.

* Studies have shown that almonds lower cholesterol by 16 points in four weeks.

* Meat and dairy products are the number one source of cholesterol.

COLDS:

There are more than 150 viruses that can cause colds. These viruses infect the upper respiratory tract and they thrive in cold temperature so it is very common to catch a cold during fall or winter. Sometimes colds are mistaken for Flu but there are very distinct differences between the two. Flu is a lot more severe with fever that ranges from 102 to 104 F. While colds very rarely develop a fever. Colds last for about a week or so but if treated in the early stages can be reduced to a few days.

In the United States $1 billion a year is wasted on nonprescription drugs for colds and coughs but often these medicines do not help the cold itself but the symptoms which are necessary tools for the body to heal itself. An example would be taking an analgesic for pain and fever such as Aspirin or Ibuprofen. Colds develop very little if any fever, a higher fever may be indication of a more serious problem. Taking these products can mask this condition. When our nose runs it is because the body is creating mucus, a secretion that traps the virus and expels it from the body. By taking an antihistamine we decrease this secretion thus keeping the virus inside. Natural remedies help the immune system fight the virus, vitamins help boost our defenses and herbs help reduce pain etc.

We recommend: At the first sign of a cold:

* Take Vitamin C and Zinc lozenges. This can help stop the cold from going through the entire process.

* Take Echinacea and goldenseal extracts. These boost the immune system.

* Put eucalyptus oil in 2 cups of boiling water and breath in the steam to help with congestion.

* Native Americans use Hyssop in tea form as an expectorant and to fight viruses.

* Gargle: A mix of water and pure tea tree oil helps sore throats.

* Drink chicken broth and potato peeling broth.

* Do not use handkerchiefs. Use paper tissues and flush them after use. The cold virus lives for several hours thus increasing the risk of reinfecting yourself.

* Wash your hands frequently to reduce the chances of re infecting yourself and others.

* Other homeopathic remedies are: Belladonna; Arsenicum; Aconite and Antimonium tartaricum.

* Take echinacea. This herb is antiviral and antibacterial, speeds healing and boosts the immune system.

* Horseradish is another herb that many use in the kitchen but also has excellent properties to treat sore throat and upper respiratory tract infections. It reduces fever and expels concentrations of mucus.

* Use kava kava as a gargle for soothing and analgesic pain relief. Helps insomnia caused by coughing and sore throat.

* Myrrh is an antiseptic and anti-inflammatory. it is very powerful and excellent for chronic sore throats. It also acts as an expectorant and decongestant and it helps cure gum disease.

* In Europe it is common to see singers use oregano oil to fight respiratory allergies, laryngitis and sore throat for it's antifungal and antibacterial properties.

* Sage is used to cure sore throat, stuffed nose, gingivitis and coughs. It is a powerful antiviral, antibacterial and antifungal. Use as a gargle.

* Wild indigo is an antiviral and antibiotic for infections. It stimulates the immune system and cures chronic sore throats.

* Mullein coats the throat with a mucus like film helping reduce the burning feeling. It clears mucus and phlegm.

* Osha is an antiviral that works great in the first stages of an infection, colds and flu, sore throat or phlegm and acts as an expectorant.

* Poke root relieves inflammation and infection and reduces coughing, pain and burning.

Make a gargle tonic with:
    1 cup of boiling water.
    2 tsp. sage leaves.
    salt.
Mix all ingredients and let them steep for 30 minutes, drain and use as gargle when needed.

Make your own cough syrup mixing:
    1 tbs. licorice root.
    1 tbs. of marshmallow root.
    1 tbs. of plantain leaves.
    1 tsp. of thyme leaf.
    4 tbs. of honey.
    4 ounces of glycerin.
    2 drops of anise oil.
Place all herbs in a container with boiling water, let it simmer for 20 minutes, strain, add honey, glycerin, and if desired, anise. Take one tbs. as needed. Keep in the refrigerator for several months.

Caution: Do not give honey to a child less than 2 years of age. It can be very harmful to them.

Cold and Flu tea.

½ tsp. echinacea root.
½ tsp. peppermint leaves.
½ tsp. hyssop leaves.
½ tsp. yarrow leaves.
½ tsp. elder flowers.
½ tsp. shizandra berries.
1 quart of boiling water.
Mix all ingredients and simmer for 30 minutes, strain and drink several cups a day.

Famous Cold remedy.

30 drops yarrow tincture.   *Do not* use if pregnant.
60 drops elderberry tincture.
20 drops peppermint leaves tincture.

4 cups of boiling water.

Add tinctures to water let it cool and drink 3 tablespoons every 4 hours.

Constipation:

Constipation refers to any irregularity in, or absence of, bowel movements. The slow movement of food through the large intestine and the amount of time the waste remains in the colon are factors that contribute to constipation. More and more water is absorbed while the waste is in our body and the stool becomes drier and bulky thus more difficult to pass.

Regular bowel movement is necessary to remove waste and toxins from the body. Some people will have movements every day; others three times a week. This is normal although some doctors consider a person moving bowels less then once a day to be constipated.

TIP: It was once believed that castor oil was a good remedy for constipation but we know now that it can cause dehydration and mineral imbalance.

Constipation can be caused by lack of exercise, too much junk food, poor diet, painkillers, antidepressants and/or pregnancy. However, serious diseases can cause constipation as well, including thyroid problems, circulatory disorder, diverticulitis, colon malfunction (fistulas, polyps, tumors, and obstruction).

TIP: Some drugs like cough syrups, codeine, blood pressure medication, calcium supplements and antihistamines can cause constipation.

In pregnant women constipation is normal due to the enlargement of the uterus pressing on the lower Intestine. It is very important to improve bowel movement while pregnant since the body is getting rid of waste and toxins coming from two persons. Do not take laxatives because they can cross the placenta barrier and cause untold damage to the baby.

Sometimes constipation can be relieved by a change in diet. Usually, people who don't eat sufficient fibers (fruits and vegetables) and don't drink enough fluids suffer from constipation.

Herbs can relieve constipation but they should be used with care. Herbal laxatives take several hours to start working, between 6 and 24 hours to be exact. If you take too much eventually the laxative will work and since too much was taken diarrhea will develop.

The following instruction will get rid of constipation. We'll teach you how to make a laxative syrup, extra strength laxatives for severe constipation and some potent herbal teas. Take any combination of the remedies in the recommended doses.

We recommend

* Take Apple pectin. It helps with constipation and brings fibers into the body.

* Take folic acid. An insufficient intake of folic acid can lead to constipation.

* To clean and heal the digestive system take, Aloe Vera juice twice a day.

* Ginger tea helps start bowel movement.

* Yerba mate in tea form is very helpful with constipation.

* Eat lots of fruits, green vegetables, cabbage, peas, carrots, garlic and sweet potatoes. All these are high in fiber.

* Exercise. Often a simple stroll in the park can relieve constipation.

* Do not take Epson salts and magnesia. Because they force the body to get rid of essential minerals.

Make a tea mixing the following:
10 boneset flowers.
10 dandelion flowers.
4 ounces of cascara bark.
2 liters of water.
Boil until reduced to half it's initial volume, add 2 tsp. of honey. Drink 2 cups a day.

Constipation relief formula.

2 tsp. cascara sagrada.
2 slices of ginger.
1 tsp. cayenne.
1 tsp. oregon grape root.
Add boiling water, let it sit for one hour. Drink 2 cups a day.

* Drink lots of water (8 glasses a day). it helps to soften stools.

* Eat prunes and drink prune juice. This is one of the best ways to relieve constipation. They act as natural laxatives. Prune juice may be the most effective and gentlest remedy for constipation.

* Cascara also known as cascara sagrada stimulates normal intestinal contractions by increasing water and salts in the bowels which tones the intestinal muscle.

* Chinese rhubarb is a stimulating laxative and purgative with astringent, cleansing effects. It does not cause excessive cramping but removes toxic bacteria from intestines and improves appetite.

* For occasional constipation use Flaxseed (also known as linseed), psyllium, or fenugreek. These herbs are concidered bulk laxatives. Flaxseed has no side effects. You can take one tablespoon of whole seeds two to three times a day followed by two cups of liquid. Drinking lots of fluid during the day is essential for these remedies to work properly.

* Dandelion root is a mild laxative good for chronic constipation. Take one tsp. of Dandelion root boiled in water three or four times a day.

Extra strength fruit and herb laxative.

½ tsp. licorice root.
½ cup of water.
3 stewed prunes.
Bring licorice root and water to a boil and simmer for 5 minutes. Remove from heat and steep for 5 minutes. Strain and add fruits, let them soak for 2 hours, eat them warm or cold as needed.

Natural laxative syrup.

1 tsp. honey.
2 tsp. cascara sagrada bark tincture.
1 tsp. licorice root tincture.
½ tsp. fennel tincture.
½ tsp. peppermint tincture.
Warm honey to liquefy it then add tinctures. Stir well and take 2 tsp. a day.

For Children:

1 tablespoon slippery elm powder and 3/4 cup water.
Combine powder and water in saucepan and heat until warm, stirring the mixture to prevent clumping. Add 2 tsp. of fruit based sweetener.

Dandruff

Dandruff occurs when skin cells renew themselves and the old cells are shed, producing irritating white flakes. Some people tend to generate and discard skin cells at a faster rate than others. Dandruff can be caused by trauma, illness, hormonal disorders, improper diet (specially the consumption of carbohydrates and sugar), deficiency of nutrients such as, B- Complex Vitamins, essential fatty acids, and selenium. Dandruff is worse during the winter. There is no cure for Dandruff, but you can minimize the condition with some powerful Natural remedies.

As we all know, it is an embarrassing problem because it is very noticeable and very itchy and sore if we do not treat it rapidly.

We recommend:

*Use flaxseed oil, primrose oil or salmon oil. They help relieve itching and inflammation. They also promote healthy skin and scalp.

*Take kelp. It improves hair growth and heals the scalp.

*Take Vitamin B complex + extra Vitamin B6 and Vitamin B12. All the B vitamins are needed to obtain a healthy skin and hair.

*Take Selenium. It is an antioxidant which aids in controlling a dry scalp.

*Take Vitamin E. It improves blood circulation.

*Take Vitamin A. It helps prevent dry skin and promote the healing of tissue.

*Take Vitamin C + Bioflavonoids. It is an important antioxidant which prevents tissue damage to the scalp and is a good healing nutrient.

*To rinse your hair use an infusion of Chaparral or Thyme. They are gentle to your hair.

Herbal conditioner for dandruff.

1 pint of water.
1 tsp. of burdock root.
1 tsp. of calendula flowers.
1 tsp. of chamomile flowers.
1 tsp. of lavender flowers.
1 tsp. of rosemary leaves.
1 tbs. of vinegar.
6 drops of sage essential oil.
Boil water and pour over herbs. Steep for 20 minutes strain and add vinegar. Apply after shampooing, do not rinse out.

*Eat a balanced diet including at least 50 to 70% of raw food.

*Avoid dairy products, fried foods, flour, chocolate, nuts, seafood and sugar.

*Make a paste mixing 8 tbs. of pure organic peanut oil and the juice of half a lemon. Before washing your hair apply the mixture and rub it into your scalp. Leave it on for 10 minutes, then shampoo your hair as usual.

*To rinse your hair use 1/4 cup of vinegar mixed with 1/4 cup of water.

*Do not pick or scratch your scalp; it only makes the dandruff worse.

*Try to use a nonoily shampoo and wash your hair frequently. Use natural products that do not have any chemicals. Every time before washing your hair massage the scalp gently with your fingers.

*Avoid using soaps, greasy ointments and creams.

*Thoroughly rub a thick gel of aloe vera leaves into the scalp; leave overnight; shampoo in the morning.

*Apple cider vinegar will help restore the proper acid/alkaline balance of the scalp and kill a bacteria that clogs the pores that release oil to the scalp. The clogged pores result in scales and crusts being formed. Apply apple cider vinegar diluted 50% with water to the scalp and let dry. There is no need to rinse. Another similar remedy suggests pouring two tablespoons into a cup, applying the straight vinegar to the scalp, and leaving it on from 15 minutes to three hours before shampooing. Lemon juice may also be used. It is the acid in these remedies that helps bring the scalp back into chemical balance.

*Rub some pure coconut oil in your hair daily. The dandruff should clear up in a few days.

*Mix 7-10 drops with the normal amount of shampoo you use. Massage into your hair and leave on for at least 2 minutes. Rinse thoroughly with water, avoiding contact with eyes. See our Product.

*Listerine For mild cases of dandruff, use the mouthwash Listerine. It has antiseptic properties. Do not use on cases where the skin is broken as the Listerine can be irritating. It used to be advertised on the back of the bottle that Listerine cures dandruff.

*Combine olive oil and ginger root and apply to your scalp before shampooing. If your dandruff is really bad, put the mixture on 10-15 minutes before shampooing.

*Rub rosemary oil or a mixture of olive oil and crushed rosemary leaves into your scalp and leave on for 15 minutes.

*Make a tea of either sage or burdock and use as a rinse after shampooing.

*Make a rinse by boiling four heaping teaspoons of dried thyme in two cups of water for ten minutes; strain and allow to cool. Massage this tea in your clean, damp hair; do not rinse out. The oil from the thyme has antiseptic properties.

* A high sugar intake may be another major cause. Sugar requires B vitamins in order to metabolize and can cause a deficiency. To compensate take a high potency B-complex to relieve the dandruff. Related to the sugar problem is the fact that diabetes may be the cause of your dandruff. If you have diabetes the high sugar levels result in dehydration of the tissues as the body flushes out fluids in an attempt to rid itself of the sugar. One of the end results is dry skin.

* Shampooing in hot water may strip out the natural oils and dry out your scalp. Using cool water will close the pores and will relieve the flaking problem.

* People on low or no fat diets may be deficient in unsaturated fats called essential fats, such as omega-3 and omega-6 fatty acids.

* Blow-drying your hair may dry out the scalp and cause dandruff. Hold your hair dryer at least 10 inches from your scalp.

Dry hair

Dry hair is a problem that develops from excessive exposure to the elements. Weather can damage and weaken the hair.
Sun, ocean water, sand, and wind dry out the scalp. Dry hair is very fragile and breaks easily especially when wet. Wet hair can stretch nearly double its length. This can be very damaging. If you have dry hair, try to brush it as little as possible when wet.

An oil treatment is recommended. This will help give your hair the natural oils that have been striped out of it and give thickness and shine. In this section you'll find a home made oil treatment for dry hair and a home made totally natural conditioner and shampoo for dry hair as well. We'll also show you how to incorporate sulfur into your diet and we'll share with you how French and Italians keep their hair healthy and shiny.

We recommend

*Use a mild shampoo containing fatty acids, protein, balsams, and moisturizers.

*Use only the amount recommended and do not repeat as this will remove too much natural oil from the hair.

*Milk and egg yolks have been used for many years to condition hair and add protein.

*Use conditioners that contain Comfrey. This herb is loaded with protein.

Essential oils for split ends.

10 drops of sandalwood essential oil.
10 drops of rosemary essential oil.
Mix the ingredients and rub them in using your fingers.

Hot oil treatment for dry hair.

2 ounces aloe vera gel.
2 ounces of castor oil.
6 drops of rose geranium cedar essential oil.
8 drops of rosemary essential oil.
2 drops of ginger essential oil.
Mix ingredients, warm oil and apply to hair and scalp in sections, cover the head with a towel and leave it on for 1 hour.
Castor oil washes easily from the hair but Italians have used olive oil for centuries.

*Garlic, onions, and all vegetables from the cabbage family are rich in sulfur.

Rinse for dry hair.

2 tsp. of comfrey essential oil.
2 tsp. of marshmallow essential oil.
2 tsp. of parsley essential oil.
2 tsp. of sage essential oil.
4 cups of water.
2 cups of vinegar.
Mix all the ingredients and use it to rinse your hair after shampooing.
Keep it away from your eyes and catch the rinse in a bowl to be used for a second and third time.

Herbal conditioner for dry hair.

1 pint of water.
1 tsp. of burdock root.
1 tsp. of calendula flowers.
1 tsp. of chamomile flowers.
1 tsp. of lavender flowers.
1 tsp. of rosemary leaves.

1 tbs. of vinegar.
Boil water and pour over herbs. Steep for 20 minutes, strain and add vinegar. Apply after shampooing. Do not rinse out.

Oily hair

If the hair contains too much oil, it becomes sticky and lifeless and the oil collects dust and dirt which makes the hair dirty. All of these things cause dandruff.

Some people have the wrong idea that if you have oily hair you need a shampoo that removes the oil from the hair. This is not the right way to treat oil excess. The solution would be to use a mild shampoo, baby shampoo is a good alternative. Most shampoos have strong chemicals that strip oil completely. This causes the oil glands in the scalp to produce even more oil.

We recommend

*Add one of these essential oils to a small amount of shampoo: cedarwood, cypress, lemon, lemongrass, sage and patchouli. These herbs reduce the oil production by the scalp.

*Avoid putting protein and balsams on your hair. This increases oiliness.

Herbal shampoo.

2 ounces unscented shampoo.
12 drops of chamomile essential oil.
12 drops of lavender essential oil.
Mix ingredients and shake well before use.

Herbal rinse for oily hair.

1 pint boiling water.
1 tsp. burdock root.
1 tsp. calendula flowers.
1 tsp. chamomile flowers.
1 tsp. lavender flowers.

1 tsp. lemongrass leaves.
1 tsp. sage leaves.
1 tbs. vinegar.
Pour water over herbs and steep for 20 minutes, strain and add vinegar. Rinse your hair with the preparation and don't rinse out.

Henna protein super preparation.

2 cups warm water.
1 egg.
1 tsp. olive oil.
2 tbs. honey.
24 drops lavender essential oil.
3 ounces henna.
Mix all the ingredients and add them to henna, removing any lumps. Wet hair and apply the preparation from root to ends cover with a plastic bag and towel to keep body heat in. This breaks down the henna and makes the color darker. Keep it covered for 1 or 2 hours. Make sure the henna does not dry out. Rinse with warm water several times, follow with shampoo and conditioner.

IMPORTANT: Use gloves and an old T-shirt to avoid staining the skin.

Dermatitis:

As we all know, the skin is the largest organ in the body and the most visible, so any condition affecting it is impossible to ignore. The skin is not only exposed to cut, burns, bruises and scrapes, it can also develop diseases just like any other part of the body.

Dermatitis or Eczema is an inflammatory skin condition that produces blisters, redness, scaling, flaking, thickening, weeping, crusting, color changes and itching that can be very annoying. Many times Dermatitis is allergic in nature mainly by coming in contact with different materials, chemicals or plants, such as, rubber, latex, perfumes, gold, silver, poison ivy, soap, cosmetics etc.

People with thin dry skin are prone to develop dermatitis and other skin conditions. Another cause of dermatitis is sensitivity or allergy to some foods. Studies have shown that people with low stomach acid are sensitive to some types of foods thus making them prone to develop some kind of skin disorder.

People suffering from dermatitis are sensitive to some of the items listed above and should be mindful of their condition and avoid contact with any irritant. Prolonged exposure to the materials may worsen the symptoms and cause the dermatitis to spread.

Another type of eczema called atopic dermatitis (AD) affects the face, elbows and knees. It's extremely itchy. Also nummular dermatitis attacks arms and legs and produces circular lesions caused by contact with nickel.

We recommend

Skin wash.

Mix the following ingredients:
1 tsp. comfrey root.
1 tsp. white oak bark.
1 tsp. slippery elm bark.
2 cups of water.
Boil for 35 minutes use it to wash the affected area.

* Vitamin B complex is needed for healthy skin.

* Taking Biotin pills is essential to prevent dermatitis.

TIP: Did you know that foods containing raw eggs prevent biotin from being absorbed?

* Put Vitamin E on the affected area. It calms the itching.

* Take Zinc orally and apply it directly to the dermatitis.

* Shark cartilage reduces inflammation.

* Use a lotion made out of blueberry leaves. This is proven to be fantastic in relieving the inflammation of dermatitis.

* Rue contains flavonoids needed for inflammation reduction.

* Drink chamomile. It helps with inflammation.

* Make a paste mixing goldenseal root powder, Vitamin E oil and honey. Apply directly on the skin. This speeds up healing.

Skin Infection fighting tea.

Make a tea mixing:
1 tsp. burdock root.
1 tsp. Oregon grape root.
1 tsp. echinacea root.
1 tsp. yellow dock root.
3 cups of water.
Boil for 20 minutes, drink ½ a cup a day.

* Do not eat the following: eggs, peanuts, wheat, dairy products, sugar, strawberries, flour.

* Use a cream made with tea tree oil. It helps kill microbes and is a natural antiseptic.

Dermatitis skin treatment.

½ pau d'arco bark tincture.
½ goldenseal root tincture.
8 drops tea tree essential oil.
8 drops chamomile essential oil.
½ cups of olive oil.
½ ounce of dried comfrey leaves.
½ ounce dried calendula flowers.
½ ounce of pure beeswax.
4 drops lavender essential oil.
Heat the olive oil with comfrey and calendula in it for about 2 hours without making the oil boil. Strain while warm, add beeswax and heat enough to melt it. Add essential oils and tinctures and stir well. Apply as needed over the skin.

＊ A very powerful herb used to treat psoriasis and dermatitis is sarsaparilla, as published in the 1940's by the New England Journal of Medicine sarsaparilla was "dramatically" successful in treating these types of conditions.

Skin Poultice.

A poultice is very helpful prepared as follows:
1 tablespoon of dried coneflower flowers.
1 tablespoon of hyssop flowers.
1 tablespoon of goldenrod flowers.
1 tablespoon of dried sunflower petals.
Mix ingredients and soak them with boiling water, let cool, place between gauze and apply on the skin, remoistening as needed.

Natural Antiseptic spray.

1/8 tsp. lemon essential oil.
1/8 tsp. tea tree essential oil.
½ ounce goldenseal tincture.
½ ounce oregon grape root tincture or barberry bark tincture.
1 ½ ounces aloe vera.
Mix all the ingredients and shake well every day for a week. Place liquid in a spray bottle, shake well before use.

＊ Studies done in France on the herbs milk thistle and gotu kola have shown that these compounds greatly improve psoriasis and dermatitis. These herbs are being used in French hospitals in the form of salve and as an injection and people in that country have used them for many years to cure leprosy.

* Licorice is a very powerful herb to reduce the inflammation, and stress related to many types of dermatitis.

* The compound gamma linoleic acid (GLA) found in primrose oil reduces inflammation of the skin better then cortisone, as shown in a study done in 100 people.

Dermatitis tea.

½ tsp. sarsaparilla root.
½ tsp. licorice root.
½ tsp. burdock root.
½ tsp. pau d'arco bark.
½ tsp. bupleurum root.
3 cups of water.
Simmer for 10 minutes and steep for another 10 minutes. Strain and drink 3 cups a day.

* Take 500 milligrams of red clover 3 times a day.

Diabetes:

Diabetes is a disease that develops due to a problem with the hormone insulin, produced by the pancreas. Insulin controls the glucose in the blood and how much glucose is absorbed by the cells; which in turn use glucose to produce energy. When insulin is not present, or the body is not using it properly, glucose can't enter the cells and stays in the bloodstream producing hyperglycemia, or excess of sugar (glucose) in the blood.

There are two types of Diabetes, Type I and type II. In type I, the pancreas produces no insulin whatsoever, therefore the patient depends on insulin injection to control the glucose. This type of diabetes affects people less than 30 years old and develops when antibodies kill cells of the pancreas in charge of creating insulin. Type II diabetes develops in people 30 years of age and older and is caused by the insufficient or ineffective production of insulin. This type of diabetes can be controlled with drugs and proper diet.

The symptoms for either type diabetes are hunger and thirst more then normal, weight loss, excessive urination, fatigue, the white part of the eye turns yellowish, one bruises easily and cuts take longer to heal.

If not managed properly diabetes can have very damaging results, such as, retinopathy, blindness, cardiovascular disease, amputation of foot or leg and kidney disease. Since Diabetes is so dangerous, it should always be monitored by a physician, but here you will learn how to manage your diabetes type II without synthetic drugs, using only herbs, vitamins and good nutrition.

Women may develop gestational diabetes during pregnancy due to the changes in the body while expecting. Although this condition disappears after delivery it is a clear sign that the woman is at risk for developing Type II diabetes later in life and is likely to suffer gestational diabetes in future pregnancies.

We recommend

* Take Alpha Lipoic Acid. It helps to control sugar level in the blood.

* Take 400 mcg. a day of Chromium Picolinate. It makes insulin more efficient helping keep sugar level low.

* Take Garlic in capsules. It helps circulation and regulates sugar level.

* 500 mg of L-glutamine and Taurine a day will reduce sugar cravings and to help release insulin.

* Take Vanadium. It helps insulin release glucose to the cells.

* Place 45 drops of ginseng tincture, 90 drops of Oregon grape root tincture and 1 ½ cups of warm water. Drink 1 cup in the course of the day.

* If you do not have high blood pressure you can take ginseng tea to lower sugar levels.

* A tea made with kidney beans, white beans, navy beans, lima beans, and northern beans removes toxins from the pancreas.

* Huckleberry promotes the production of insulin.

* Take Dandelion root to protect the liver.

* Eat Jupiter berries. They lower blood sugar levels.

* Eat a well-balanced diet, rich in fibers (raw vegetables and fruits).

TIP: Did you know that carrots raise blood sugar levels more than ice cream?

* If you are planning to get pregnant, be sure to control your diabetes months before you start trying. Should you become pregnant before it's managed, the baby could have birth defects in the first few weeks of pregnancy.

* Take good care of your feet. If you have diabetes, the nerves of the foot are the first part to get damaged, losing the sensation of

pain; this is the main reason for foot amputation in people with diabetes.

* Wear comfortable shoes, with white cotton socks, keep them dry.

* If your child has diabetes make sure that his or her teacher knows exactly what the symptoms are, and what to do in case of poglycemia (too little glucose in the blood) and hyperglycemia (too much glucose in the blood).

Diarrhea:

When stools are loose and without consistency it is called diarrhea, an effective way for the body to get rid of an undesirable substance. This may be followed with symptoms like vomiting, stomach pain, thirst, fever, nausea and/or dehydration. In children and people 65 and older this may be dangerous.

Diarrhea and vomiting cause the loss of fluids which need to be replaced. In some cases diarrhea is the secondary symptom of another problem, but in most instances it is caused by food poisoning; bacteria in food or water; food allergies; or a virus. Also, excess alcohol consumption, laxatives and caffeine are known to cause diarrhea. Some medicines can trigger diarrhea, such as antibiotics (tetracycline, clyndamycin, penicillin). If you find, blood or mucus in the stool that is a sign of infection or parasites.

Some well known drugs will stop diarrhea but they interfere with the natural process of cleansing that the body desperately needs. With natural remedies we may help ourselves feel better without stopping the immune system from doing its job.

Your body uses diarrhea to flush bacteria or viruses you might have ingested by eating bad food. Therefore, it might be a bad idea to stop diarrhea too quickly. However, diarrhea does not work sometimes and if goes on for several days, dehydration and loss of important nutrients may occur which can be dangerous, especially in children. That's why we recommend the use of herbs instead of over the counter drugs. Using herbs you can stop diarrhea and target the cause of it at the same time.

FACT: The use of the vaccine against rotavirus has been stopped by the National Centers for Disease Control and Prevention and FDA for causing bowel obstruction.

We recommend:

* Take homeopathic Arsenicum if you feel you have eaten spoiled food. This will help control the discharge without interfering with the elimination of toxins.

* If you feel weak and have a burning pain in mid-section take cuprum arsenicosum .
Take 4 charcoal tablets every hour this will absorb the toxins from the body.

* Drink blackberry tea for mild diarrhea.

* Take cayenne in capsules.

* Wild oregano oil is an antibacterial, anti parasitic and anti viral.

* Ginger tea can stop cramps and pain.

* Drink plenty of fluids, but stay away from caffeine and alcohol. Drinks like ginger ale or carrot juice are good for making the stools less watery.

> TIP: Do not drink apple juice this will make diarrhea worse.

* Boil brown rice and water for 45 minutes eat the rice (it contains Vitamin B) and drink the water.

* Do not eat dairy products. When suffering from diarrhea the body loses the enzyme needed to digest lactose.

* The homeopathic remedy Sulfur is excellent for diarrhea.

* Take charcoal tablets every 4 hours to absorb toxins.

Blackberry remedy.

1 tbs. chamomile tincture.
1/4 cup of blackberry brandy.
3 drops of ginger essential oil.
2 drops of peppermint essential oil.
Mix ingredients and shake well. Take 1 tablespoon every hour.

Blueberry remedy.

4 tbs. of dried blueberries.
1 pint of water.
Mix and boil the ingredients, simmer for 20 minutes, strain and drink 4 tablespoons every hour.

Traveler's remedy.

1 ounce quassia bark tincture.
1 ounce goldenseal root tincture.
½ ounce yerba santa leaves tincture.
½ ounce peppermint leaves tincture.
Mix this very bitter remedy and take 1 teaspoon 30 minutes before meals as a preventive treatment. If already ill, double the dose.

Diarrhea Remedies for children.

Children develop diarrhea frequently and the causes sometimes are different from those of adults. A child could suffer a bout of diarrhea simply by eating too fast, too much, or by eating foods that are too difficult for the young to digest. Also, intestinal flu and intolerance to some intestinal bacteria can cause diarrhea in children.

For adults, is ok to use blackberry root but for children this can be too potent. Instead the berries or leaves of the plant can be used to stop diarrhea in children but make sure to remove the seeds as they can act as a laxative which is the opposite result.

Children diarrhea tea.

3 cups of water.
1 tsp. catnip leaves.
½ tsp. raspberry or blackberry leaves.
½ tsp. slippery elm bark.
½ tsp. peppermint leaves.
½ tsp. cinnamon bark powder.
Mix ingredients and simmer for 5 minutes, remove from heat and steep for 20 minutes, strain and give several times a day.

Blackberry shake.

½ cup blackberry juice.
1 banana.
½ tsp. cinnamon bark powder.
1 tsp. sugar.
Blend in all ingredients, and serve. Your child will love it.

Rice preparation for diarrhea.

½ cup of rice.
2 cups of water.
1/4 tsp. oregon grape root powdered.
½ tsp. cinnamon powder.
1 banana.
Boil rice and water until soft, (30 minutes). Blend rice oregon root powder and banana. Serve and sprinkle cinnamon on top. Rice and banana help stop diarrhea and return important nutrients lost.

Eye problems:

The eyes are two of the most complicated organs in the human body. They are a very important part of our day to day life and there are several conditions that can affect the eyes. We all have experienced at one time or another some type of eye problem such as irritation, dryness, red eye, or some more serious conditions like cataract or blindness.

Although most of the time eye problems are localized or within the eye itself, the eyes also reflect diseases elsewhere in the body; for example blured vision can be a sign of diabetes, yellow eyes can be a clue to hepatitis and a marked difference in the pupil's size can indicate that a tumor is developing somewhere in the body.

We take for granted the power of vision and the complexity of the whole process. The eye ball is a sphere measuring about one inch in diameter coated with a white substance called sclera commonly known as the "white of the eye". Under the sclera is a network of blood vessels called choroid.
The part of the eye that we see from outside is covered with the cornea and in the center is the iris which can have several different colors. It gives us our eye pigmentation or "eye color". In the center of the iris is the pupil which is in charge of letting light inside the eye. Behind the iris (going inside the eye) are the lens and the retina which are sensitive to the light let in by the pupil. The retina is connected to the optic nerve and this one is connected to the brain.

There are six muscles outside the eye in charge of moving the eye (left, right, up and down) and other muscles inside the eye are in charge of focusing the lens so you can see far away or closer. There are also fluids that fill the eyeball and lubricants called tears that clean and protect the front of the eye.
But how does everything work? The action of seeing something is very complex and amazingly fast. First, light enters the eye through the pupil which contracts and expands depending on the amount of light in the environment.

We need light in order to see, therefore, the pupil expands in darkness to allow more light to go in the eye. When too much light is in the environment, the pupil contracts to let less light in. As it enters the eye, the lens focuses light by thickening or thinning its size. Once focused, the light is transferred to the retina which in turn builds an image by using pigments. After the image is formed, it's sent through the optic nerve to the brain where the image is interpreted and analyzed.

To all this we have to add the other eye and the work that is performed by both eyes together which gives us the ability to see and judge distances, speed and movement so obviously these organs are very complex and important and any interference, in any of the steps mentioned, can result in a vision problem.

Many eye conditions can be prevented with proper diet and herbs.

Conjunctivitis

Conjunctivitis or "pink eye" is an inflammation of the conjunctiva which is the membrane that covers the entire eyeball and the inside of the eyelids. The symptoms of conjunctivitis are redness, eye pain, burning, blured vision, feeling of dryness and discharge of a sticky fluid.
Conjunctivitis is very contagious. Wash your hands and do not touch the affected area.

We recommend

Mix 2 tsp. chamomile flowers.
1 tsp. Oregon grape root.
2 cups of boiling water.
Let it sit for 20 minutes, cool, strain and use an eyewash.

* Use calendula in bacterial or viral conjunctivitis to reduce itching and inflammation, heal and soothe. It's an antiseptic perfect for irritation due to pollutants and allergies. Use it as a local compress and eyewash. It is available in eye drops as well.

* Use a lotion made out of Vitamin A and apply it directly.

* If the eye is swollen, peel a potato, cut it in thin slices and place them on eyes affected by conjunctivitis.

* Use Fennel. This plant although used in the kitchen for salads is also a very good herb for vision problems. When snakes shed their skin they are temporarily blinded and eat fennel to restore their sight. It can be eaten raw or made as a tea and the tea can be used as an eyewash.

* Use Eyebright herb in drops. It's excellent for conjunctivitis. This plant can be used internally and is much more effective than commercial eye drops and safer.

* Goldenseal is an anti inflammatory and natural antibiotic. It kills many different kinds of bacteria and decreases swelling by removing fluid from tissues.

* Make a tea with goldthread. It treats inflammation of the conjunctiva and infection of eyes. It's also a good pain reliever. The tea can be use as an eyewash.

BACK

Bloodshot eyes

A bloodshot eye is a condition that develops when the small blood vessels that we see on the surface of the eye become inflamed with too much blood caused by insufficient oxygen to the cornea.
If overwhelmed with fatigue, eyestrain, alcohol consumption, insufficient Vitamin B2 and B6 or high blood pressure, bloodshot eyes may appear. However if all of these conditions are managed, bloodshot eyes should disappear.

We recommend

* Vitamin A is very necessary for a healthy vision.

* Eat spinach and take Lutein or spinach extract because they contain carotenoid needed for retina and eye tissue.

* Take a Vitamin B complex. About 100 mg. of each B vitamin 3 times a day has been shown to releive the B vitamin deficiency that leads to bloodshot eyes.

* Use raspberry leaves to make a tea and when cool, soak a piece of cotton and apply it to the eye.

* Using Eyebright herb in drops is excellent for bloodshot eyes. This plant can be use internally and is much more effective than commercial eye drops and safer.

* Cayenne it's an anti inflammatory for the mucus membranes Use very small amounts well diluted or in an eye drop form.

* Take Ginkgo biloba. It increases the delivery of oxygen and nutrients to the eye.

BACK

Cataracts

Cataracts are a clouding of the eye lens that causes blured vision, inability to focus and is progressive and painless. The cataract becomes thicker with time until it blinds the eye and is the number one cause of blindness in the world.
The most common type of cataract is senile cataract which means that it affects people 65 and older. This type of cataract is caused by free radicals that damage the lens.

TIP: Frequent x-ray causes the formation of chemical reactive fragments in the eye and this leads to cataracts

We recommend

Mix 1 cup of rose petals.
4 tbsp. of raspberry leaves.
4 cups of boiling water.
Let the ingredients rest for 30 minutes, strain and use as eye wash.

* Using Eyebright herb in drops is excellent for cataracts. This plant can be used internally and is much more effective than commercial eye drops and safer.

* Eat spinach and take Lutein or spinach extract because they contain carotenoid needed for retina and eye tissue and sometimes reverses cataracts.

* Vitamin A is very necessary for a healthy vision.

* Dusty miller is used to dissolve cataracts and corneal opacities if used in the early stages of the disease.

* Take Ginkgo biloba because it increases the delivery of oxygen and nutrients to the eye and clears toxins.

* Eat lots of green vegetables, especially spinach and, kale as well as berries, blueberries, blackberries, cherries and fruits rich in Vitamin C and E.

* Avoid dairy products and saturated fats as these produce free radicals which cause cataracts and damage to the lens.

* Do not use any antihistamines if you have cataracts.

* Bilberry Strengthens and protects veins and blood vessels, protects the retina, reduces pressure in glaucoma and can stop the growth of cataracts.

BACK

Glaucoma

Glaucoma is a very serious disease that affects the optic nerve. The pressure inside the eye rises, damaging the nerve and causing vision loss and blindness. People more than 65 years of age are at risk and people with diabetes as well.
This condition produces no symptoms. Therefore, people who suffer glaucoma do not find out until it's very advanced.
Glaucoma has probably many causes. Some scientists claim It Is related to stress, poor nutrition and high blood pressure. Collagen deficiency has been linked to glaucoma.

We recommend

* Take 50 mg. of Rutin 3 times a day. This bioflavonoid reduces pain and pressure inside the eye.

* Vitamin A and carotenoid are needed to keep healthy eyes and to improve night vision.

* Eat spinach and take Lutein or spinach extract because they contains carotenoid needed for retina and eye tissue and sometimes reverses many eye conditions.

* Eyebright herb in drops is excellent for glaucoma. This plant can be use internally and is much more effective than commercial eye drops and safer.

* Take Ginkgo Biloba because it increases the delivery of oxygen and nutrients to the eye and it clears toxins. Mix it with zinc sulfate to slow down progressive vision loss.

* Cayenne is an anti inflammatory for the mucus membranes. Use very small amounts, well diluted with water or in eye drop form. It increases blood flow to the eye.

* Take Vitamin E. It removes particles from the eye lens.

* Bilberry strengthens and protects veins and blood vessels, protects the retina, reduces pressure in glaucoma and can stop the growth of cataracts.

* Use Coleus dropped directly into the eye to increase blood flow to the eye and decrease intraocular pressure.

* Use Fennel. This plant although used in the kitchen for salads is also a very good herb for vision problems. When snakes shed their skin they are temporarily blinded and eat fennel to restore their sight. It can be eaten raw or made as a tea and the tea can be used as an eyewash.

* Jaborandi is a herb that grows in the rainforest. It's been used for about 120 years in patients with glaucoma because it contains pilocarpine.

* Although we do not recommend it, many studies have shown that marijuana can help reduce intraocular pressure but it is unknown how marijuana achieves this result.

BACK

Diabetic retinopathy

Diabetes can cause retinopathy, a condition that develops when tinny blood vessels connected to the retina begin to leak. Then more blood vessels grow in the affected area causing vision problems and blindness in thousands of people suffering diabetes. Since this disease causes no symptoms in the beginning it is very hard to diagnose until the condition is advanced.

We recommend

* Vitamin A and carotenoid are needed to keep healthy eyes and to improve night vision.

* Take Ginkgo Biloba to increase the delivery of oxygen and nutrients to the eye and to clear toxins. It is very helpful in retinopathy.

* Bilberry strengthens and protects veins and blood vessels, protects the retina, reduces pressure in glaucoma and damage cause by diabetic retinopathy.

* Grape seed extract contains procyanidins which strengthens retinal capillaries and prevents clots or bleeding, provides vital nutrients, increases night vision and slows eye ageing. It also prevents and treats retinopathy and arteriosclerosis in the eye.

* Eat spinach and take Lutein or spinach extract. They contain carotenoid needed for retina and eye tissue and sometimes reverses many eye conditions.

* We recommend that you check Diabetes for important herbs and nutrients needed for diabetes and to prevent diabetic retinopathy.

Fever:

Fever is an elevation in body temperature. It's the body's protective mechanism against infection. The elevation in temperature happens when our immune system is fighting off bacteria and viruses that could harm our body. Fever is our strongest weapon in the fight against infections or diseases.

Normal body temperature ranges from 97 to 99 degrees Fahrenheit but varies throughout the day. Usually it's lower in the early morning and higher in late afternoon. A fever is considered to be any temperature above 100 degrees Fahrenheit. One should be concerned when temperature rises above 102 degrees Fahrenheit for an adult and 103 degrees Fahrenheit for children.

Often, having a high temperature is helpful for the body; it's the way the body acts to destroy harmful microbes. In an adult temperature less than 103 degrees Fahrenheit encourage the body to create more immune cells. A fever of 104 or higher can be a risk for people with cardiac problems since it accelerates the heart beat making it work harder and can cause irregular rhythms, chest pain or even heart attack. When a person has had a fever of more than 106 degrees for a long period of time it can cause dehydration and brain damage.

Although vigorous exercise in which the muscles generate heat faster than the body can dissipate it can cause a temporary rise in temperature it is not considered fever.

We recommend:

* Drink as much water as you can in order to replace fluid loss. It will also help bring down body temperature.

* Rest as much as possible.

* Avoid sudden changes in atmospheric temperatures.

* Avoid eating solid foods until the fever is gone. You can replace the foods by drinking plenty of distilled water and/or juices.

* When you have fever do not take any supplement containing either iron or zinc. Taking iron causes great tension in a body that is fighting infection and zinc is not absorbed by the body when you have fever.

* Take cool baths. Fill a bath tub, submerge and lie down for approximately 5 minutes. Repeat as needed until the fever is down.

* If the fever does not exceed 102 degrees let it run its course. It helps the body fight infection and eliminate toxins.

* When a child has fever do not give them aspirin. Instead try to reduce the fever with cold baths.

* If a baby of 3 months or younger has 103 degrees or more, call your doctor. If a child with fever has also a stiff neck, swelling of the throat or disorientation, see a physician immediately as these symptoms may indicate meningitis.

* To reduce fever some beneficial herbs include Blackthorn, Echinacea, Fenugreek seed, Feverfew, Ginger and Poke root. Caution: Avoid Feverfew during pregnancy.

* Taking a tea or a hot steam bath made with Elderberry may help.

* If you develop an unusually high fever, sponge your face and forehead with lukewarm water. It will reduce the fever and you will feel more comfortable.

To reduce fever you can make this tea:
1 tsp. Echinacea root.
1 tsp. White willow root.
1 cup water.
Combine ingredients in a pan, cover and bring to a boil. Reduce heat and simmer for 30 minutes, cool and strain. Take half a cup up to 4 times a day.

Flu :

Influenza, most commonly know as "the flu" or "grippe", is caused by a virus that infects the upper respiratory tract. There are two types of influenza, type A and B. They infect the throat, nose, lungs bronchial tubes, and middle ear. There are vaccines for the flu but since there are so many viruses that can cause influenza (about 200) they are constantly mutating, making it very difficult to achieve success against these types of viruses.
The symptoms for influenza are similar to those of a common cold, body aches, cough, hot and cold sweat, fatigue, headaches, fever, nausea, vomiting, throat pain and lack of appetite. Colds last for a week but the flu can last for up to 12 days and after all symptoms have disappeared a persistent cough remains for another week.
Influenza is one of the thousands of diseases that modern medicine has yet to find a cure for but herbs and natural remedies can relieve the symptoms.

TIP: Did you know that the Flu shot or vaccine is made from chicken embryos? If you are allergic to eggs avoid Flu shots.
The allergic reaction is worse then the flu symptoms. Besides, the effectiveness of the vaccine is not very good either.

Do not buy any over the counter drugs to deal with this virus. Most of the medications on the market today only suppress the symptoms and block the self defense mechanism of the body making it more difficult to recover.

TIP: Do not use Aspirin. This can irritate the mucus membranes.

We recommend

* Take Vitamin C to boost immune system and increase the number of white blood cells.

* Take Zinc lozenges to boost the immune system as soon the symptoms develop.

* Colloidal silver kills viruses.

* Take Garlic capsules to decrease the growth of the virus.

Make a tea mixing:

1 tsp. bayberry bark.
1 tsp. grated ginger root.
½ tsp. cayenne powder.
1 cup of boiling water.
Let it sit for 20 minutes.

* Take "cold and flu" tablets. This homeopathic preparation has helped people avoid getting infected with the flu virus by taking one tablet a day throughout the flu season.

* Arsenicum album is a great homeopathic remedy. Take it if you are thirsty but feel better drinking warm fluids, lack of appetite, body aches, and feel worse during the night.

* Take bryonia if you cough or have throat and chest pain, dry mouth and lips or are very thirsty.

* Take eupatorium perfoliatum if you have pain in your bones and eyeballs.

* Take Gelsemium if you have chills, aches, fever but are not thirsty.

* Nux vomica is used when a simple cold has developed into influenza.

* If the fever is too high, take catnip tea and ½ tsp. of lobeliatincture every 4 hours. Do not use if pregnant or breast-feeding and do not give to a child less than one year old.

* Cat's claw shortens the duration of the flu.

* Cayenne in powder form added to juice or soup is very helpful for cleaning of mucus from the system and for relieving congestion.

* For cough, place echinacea extract (alcohol free) and goldenseal in your mouth and hold it for a few minutes, then swallow. This will keep the virus from multiplying.

* Elderberry it's an antiviral.

* Take a very warm bath with eucalyptus oil in the water. This will relieve your congestion.

* Olive leaf extract kills all types of viruses including the flu virus.

* Drink lots of juices and eat chicken soup to avoid dehydration.

* Take echinacea. This herb is antiviral and antibacterial and speeds healing and boosts the immune system.

* Horseradish is another herb that many use in the kitchen but it also has excellent properties to treat sore throat and upper respiratory tract infections. It reduces fever and expels concentrations of mucus.

* Use kava kava as a gargle for soothing and analgesic pain relief. Helps insomnia caused by coughing and sore throat.

* Myrrh is an antiseptic and anti-inflammatory, very powerful and excellent for chronic sore throats. It acts also as an expectorant and decongestant. It helps cure gum disease.

* In Europe it is common to see singers use oregano oil to fight respiratory allergies, laryngitis and sore throat. They take it for it's antifungal and antibacterial properties.

* Sage is used to cure sore throat, stuffed nose, gingivitis and coughs. It is a powerful antiviral, antibacterial and antifungal. Use as a gargle.

* Wild indigo is an antiviral and antibiotic for infections. It stimulates the immune system and cures chronic sore throats.

* Mullein coats the throat with a mucus-like film which helps reduce the burning feeling. It clears mucus and phlegm.

* Osha is an antiviral that works great in the first stages of the infection of colds and flu, sore throat and phlegm. It acts as an expectorant.

* Poke root relieves inflammation and infection. It reduces coughing, pain and burning.

Make a gargle tonic with:
   1 cup of boiling water.
   2 tsp. sage leaves.
   salt.
Mix all ingredients and let them steep for 30 minutes, drain and use as gargle when needed.

Make your own cough syrup mixing:

   1 tbsp. licoriceroot.
   1 tbsp. of marshmallow root.
   1 tbsp. of plantain leaves.
   1 tsp. of thyme leaf.

4 tbsp. of honey.

4 ounces of glycerin.

2 drops of anise oil.

Place all herbs in a container with boiling water, let it simmer for 20 minutes, strain, add honey, glycerin and, if desired, anise. Take 1 tbsp. as needed. It will keep in the refrigerator for several months.

Caution: Do not give honey to a child less than 2 years of age. It can be very harmful to them.

Gallbladder Disorders

The gallbladder is a 3 to 4 inch-long pear-shaped organ located on the right side of the body, directly under the liver. One of the functions of the liver is to remove poisonous substance from blood so that they can be excreted from the body. The liver excretes all these gathered toxins in a digestive agent called bile. Bile also contains cholesterol, bile salts, lecithin, and other substances. The bile (about one pint of it every day) goes first to the gallbladder, which holds it until food arrives in the small intestine. The gallbladder then releases the bile, which passes through cystic and bile ducts into the small intestine. Ultimately, the toxins are passed out of the body through the feces.

Abnormal concentration of bile acids, cholesterol and phospholipids in the bile can cause the formation of gallstones. The presence of gallstones is known to doctors as cholelithiasis. It has been estimated that 20 million Americans have gallstones. In fact, one in ten people have gallstones without knowing it. However, if a stone is pushed out of the gallbladder and lodges in the bile duct, this can cause nausea, vomiting, and pain in the upper right abdominal region. These symptoms often arise after the individual has eaten fried or fatty foods.

Gallstones can range from the size of a tiny grain of sand to larger than a pea-sized mass. Seventy five percent of gallstones are cholesterol stones, with the remaining 25 percent being pigment stones. Pigment stones are composed of calcium salts. Although the cause of pigment stones is unknown, factors such as intestinal surgery, cirrhosis of the liver, and blood disorders can increase the rate risk.

The presence of gallstones creates a possibility that cystitis, inflammation of the gallbladder, may develop. This can cause severe pain in the upper right abdomen and/or across the chest, possibly accompanied of fever, nausea, and vomiting. Other symptoms of gallbladder disease include constant pain below the breastbone that shoots into the right or left shoulder and radiates into the back. The pain can last from 30 minutes to several hours. The urine may be tea- or coffee-colored, and there may be shaking, chills, and a yellowish discoloration of the skin and eyes. Gallbladder attacks occur often in the evening and can take place sporadically. Abdominal pain that occurs on a daily basis may be a problem unrelated to the gallbladder. A gallbladder attack may mimic a heart attack, with severe pain in the chest area.

Inflammation of the gallbladder requires immediate treatment. If left untreated, it can be life threatening.

I recommend

- Alfalfa cleanses the liver and supplies necessary vitamins and minerals. Twice a day for two days, take 1,000 milligrams in tablet or capsule form with a glass of warm water.

- Peppermint capsules are used in Europe to cleanse the gallbladder.

- If you have gallstones, or are prone to developing them, turmeric can reduce your risk of further problems.

- Other beneficial herbs include barberry root bark, catnip, cramp bark, dandelion, fennel, ginger root, horsetail, parsley and wild yam. DO NOT USE BARBERRY DURING PREGNANCY.

- If you have an attack, drink 1 tablespoon of apple cider in a glass of apple juice. This should relieve the pain quickly. If the pain does not subside, go to the emergency room to rule out other disorders such as gastroesophogeal reflux disease or heart problems.

Hair loss:

In general, hair loss is a condition that reflects the level of health of the person. Although not a dangerous disease, millions of people are desperately seeking a cure for hair loss. Our society drives us to look healthy and young and hair loss damages our looks and our self esteem, making us less sure of ourselves.

But why do some people suffer from hair loss and others enjoy a full head of hair throughout their lives? Usually we lose about 100 hairs per day after a few months, a new hair grows out of the same follicle. In some men the new hair is thinner than the one before and when this one falls the next one is even thinner until eventually the follicle stops producing hair.

Women also suffer from hair loss as they age and reach menopause although they don't lose as much hair as men. Childbirth can cause hair loss. Mothers usually lose a lot of hair during a 6-month period after giving birth. Other reasons for hair loss in men and women are; stress, infection, surgery, high fever, diets, over brushing, syphilis and tumors.

There are some drugs that claim to regrow hair but they only achieve mild results and are full of side effects, for example minoxidil (Rogaine) should not be taken by people with high blood pressure and it may cause acne on the forehead and back. Another is finasteride (Propecia) which can be taken orally (men only) and causes sex problems, rash and if handled by a pregnant woman, can cause birth defects in the genital area of the fetus.

We recommend

TIP: Did you know that the herb Sage used as a rinse restores color to gray hair better then advertised products?

* Take Vitamins A, B6, B12, Folic acid, biotin, and Vitamin C. Caution:Too much Vitamin A can cause hair loss keep your intake less than 100,000 IU daily.

* Take Silica in capsules once a day to make hair stronger and thicker.

* Rinse your hair with a mix of apple cider vinegar and sage tea to help hair grow.

* To improve blood circulation to the scalp take Ginkgo Biloba.

* Take Saw Palmetto herb to unblock hair follicles and heal the prostate (like the drug found in Rogaine) by decreasing residues of dihydrotestosterone (DHT) in the scalp. It is 3 times more effective then Proscar in healing the prostate. It may be 3 times better then Rogaine.

* Nettles can be used locally or internally to prevent baldness and stimulate hair growth because it contains high amounts of silica.

* Use Rosemary oil locally to stimulate hair growth. It improves oxygen delivery to the follicles.

* Neem has been used in ayurveda for hundreds of years to help hair growth. It thickens hair, heals follicles and cleans the scalp.

* Horsetail contains silica therefore promoting hair growth.

* A Chinese herb called Fo-Ti restores hair color and hinders production of DHT, stops hair loss and thinning hair and encourages hair growth.

* Tea tree oil kills bacteria and mites that attack the follicles and causes hair loss.

Mix 1 tsp. of cayenne.
    1 tsp. of yucca root.
    2 cups of boiling water.
Let it sit for 30 minutes then apply this topical solution on the scalp to promote blood circulation to the area and help prevent hair loss.

* Pygeum works in the same way Saw palmetto does by reducing DHT in the scalp and thus promoting hair growth.

* Avoid drugs such as Rogaine and Propecia. They have side effects and although they are allowed to advertise that they re grow hair, only a small percentage of people see acceptable results. Besides, they must be used for the rest of your life. As soon as you stop, the

hair loss resumes and some people have reported loss of hair at a higher pace then before the treatment started.

* Use shampoos and conditioners containing silica and biotin extracts.

* Avoid hair sprays and gels.

* Do not brush your hair too much.

* When towel drying your hair, don't rub. Instead pat your hair dry gently.

Rosemary Hair Oil.

1/2 tsp. rosemary essential oil.
1/2 tsp. jojoba oil.
Mix ingredients in a blender and process until smooth. Apply on the scalp a leave it for a few hours before washing it off.

Hair Formula.

1 cup aloe vera gel.
4 tbs. apple cider vinegar.
1 tbs. nettle tincture.
1/2 tsp. vitamin E oil.
1/2 tsp. rosemary essential oil.
Mix ingredients in a blender and process until smooth. Apply a small amount on the scalp once a day.

Hemorrhoids:

Hemorrhoids are swollen anal varicose veins. These veins can become so stretched that they push with extreme force, then rupture and bleed. The hemorrhoids cause rectal bleeding, pain, burning, inflammation, irritation and itching since the swollen tissues are difficult to keep clean.

Hemorrhoids may be external or internal. The external hemorrhoids you can see and feel as a soft bluish-purple lump. The internal hemorrhoids you probably won't notice because they are usually painless. There is another type of hemorrhoid called prolapsed, it is an internal hemorrhoid that collapses and protrudes outside the anus accompanied by a mucus discharge and heavy bleeding. They can become thrombosed and are terribly painful. The most common cause of hemorrhoids is chronic constipation or congested liver.

Other factors that can cause or contribute to hemorrhoids include obesity, poor exercise, food allergies, lifting heavy objects and insufficient consumption of dietary fiber.

In pregnancy, women can develop hemorrhoids due to the pressure of the growing uterus on the mayor veins. Constipation in pregnancy can make hemorrhoids more painful. Straining during bowel movement puts a lot of pressure on the veins around the anus area. Hemorrhoids are also common after childbirth.

We recommend:

* Eat foods that are high in dietary fiber, like wheat bran, fruits and vegetables. Also eat apples, broccoli, carrots, Brazil nuts, green beans, guar gum, lima beans, oat bran, pears, beets, peas, whole grains, psyllium seed and foods In the cabbage family. It's the best treatment to prevent and treat hemorrhoids.

* To help bleeding hemorrhoids eat foods highs in Vitamin K, such as alfalfa, dark green leafy vegetables and black strap molasses.

* Drink plenty of fluids to help prevent constipation. Fluids are the best stool softener.

* Avoid fats, animal products, coffee, alcohol and hot spices. They are hard on the lower digestive tract.

* Take flaxseed oil daily. It helps soften stools. Take 1 or 2 tbsp. in the morning.

* Do not strain when moving the bowels. Do not sit on the toilet for more than 10 minutes at a time to prevent the blood from pooling in the hemorrhoidal veins.

* Take a hot bath for 15 minutes to help reduce swelling and ease pain. Do not add bath beads, oils or bubbles. They can irritate sensitive tissues.

* Avoid cleaning the anus with soap. It can cause irritation to the affected area.

* Do not sit on hard surfaces. That can make hemorrhoids more painful.

* When you lift any object, do not hold your breath. That puts enormous strain and pressure upon the hemorrhoidal vessels.

* Do not use rough toilet paper. Instead use baby wipes or a moistened toilet paper.

* Avoid sitting or standing for long periods of time.

* Apply Aloe Vera gel directly on the anus. It relieves pain and soothes the burning sensation.

* Use Bayberry, goldenseal root, myrrh, and white oak in a salve form to relieve pain in the hemorrhoids.

* Brew a strong, warm tea using Lady's mantle (yarrow) and apply it to the hemorrhoids with a cotton ball several times a day or as required.

* Apply Witch hazel with a sterile cotton pad 3 times daily to shrink the swollen veins.

* Take Buck thorn bark, collinsonia root, parsley, red grape vine leaves or stone root either in capsules or tea form. They are also good for the treatment of hemorrhoids.

* To keep the bowels clean use Cayenne (capsicum) or garlic enemas. They relieve pain caused by hemorrhoids.

* To help heal hemorrhoids use a peeled clove of garlic 3 times a week as a suppository. Or peel a raw potato and cut it into a small cone shaped piece and follow the same procedure.

* Take an infusion of Pilewort. If it doesn't help, in addition drink a tea made of Witch Hazel, Periwinkle or Tormentil. Also, you can apply Pilewort ointment on the affected area 2 or 3 times a day.

* Take Butcher's Broom. It reduces inflammation and helps increase circulation. Use also externally to reduce swelling.

* Use Comfrey as an ointment, powdered root or tea from the leaf or powder to soothe irritation. It also promotes healing of tissues and is an anti-inflammatory.

* Use Horse Chestnut. It shrinks hemorrhoids, reduces swelling, pain and itching. It also strengthens blood vessels, tones the veins and is an anti-inflammatory.

* Apply Mullein flower or infusion in the hemorrhoids to speed tissue healing. It is a soothing emollient for dry, sore and irritated hemorrhoids.

* Use Peony. It helps with burning, itching or irritated hemorrhoids or pain after stools. It also helps repair fissures, ulcers and fistula.

* Apply Plantain ointments directly on the hemorrhoid to relieve irritation and swelling. it shrinks swollen veins and decreases bleeding.

* Use Stone root. it relieves pain, itching and burning of chronic protruding or internal hemorrhoids. it also reduces bleeding and helps with chronic diarrhea or constipation.

* To reduce inflammation and encourage healing, make a small Witch Hazel compress and keep it on the affected area for as long as possible.

* Add Bayberry and Yellow dock (both astringent herbs) and add them to cocoa butter which can then be shaped into a suppository and placed in the anus.

* Make this tea or wash for hemorrhoids to relieve pain and help the affected area heal faster.
1 tsp. evening primrose
1 tsp. self- heal
1 tsp. peppermint leaves
1/4 water
Combine all the ingredients in a pan and boil until the liquid is reduced to 2 cups, then strain. Drink up to 2 cups a day.

Hemorrhoids Wash.
1 tsp. Blackberry leaves
1 tsp. Witch hazel leaves
1 tsp. mullein
2 cups boiling water
Combine all the ingredients in a nonmetallic container and cover with the boiling water, steep for 30 minutes, cool and strain. Use as wash whenever needed.

* Supplements are also important to prevent or cure hemorrhoids. Supplements such as:

Calcium + Magnesium. It help prevent cancer of the colon and is essential for blood clotting.

Vitamin C + bioflavonoids with hesperidin and rutin speed healing.

Vitamin B complex + Vitamin B12 + choline and inositol reduce stress on the rectum and improve digestion.

Coenzyme Q10 helps heal faster and increases cellular oxygenation.

Potassium prevents constipation which can cause hemorrhoids.

Shark cartilage treats pain and inflammation.

Vitamin D3 aids in the healing of mucous membranes and tissues. It helps to absorb calcium.

* Here are some homeopathic remedies to cure hemorrhoids.

If the hemorrhoids are accompanied by aching in the lower back and at the base of the spine or a sensation in the rectum like splinters or sticks or a sensation of pressure in the rectum as if would protrude and there is little or no bleeding take Aesculus.

If you have a mild discomfort such as stinging pains, tight sensation or a constant uneasy feeling in the anal area which is worse in the morning, wearing tight clothes or is worse in cold or open air and there is a little or no bleeding or if you have itching in the anus and if you apply cold water you feel relief or you have chronic constipation, take Nux vomica. Also if the hemorrhoids appeared after overuse of laxatives, coffee, medications or drugs, take Nux vomica.

When itching is the predominant symptom or you have a burning or sore pain in the rectum and you feel better when applying cold water and you have diarrhea rather than constipation, take Aloe.

This remedy is ideal during the first 2 days of acute inflammation around the hemorrhoids. If you have too much redness and swelling and great pain and tenderness in the hemorrhoids, take Belladonna.

* If you can barely stand a very light touch on the inflamed hemorrhoid or if you see blood during a bowel movement and it feels better when applying warm water, take Muriatic acid.

* If you see a significant amount of dark, thick blood flow from the hemorrhoids and they are not tender to touch and you feel pulsation in the rectum, take Hamamelis.

* If you find relief applying cold pads and you feel thirst less and you don't want any clothes touching the hemorrhoids plus no two stools are alike in color or consistency, take Pulsatilla.

Caution: All the homeopathic remedies listed can be used by pregnant women, except Hamamelis.

Insomnia:

Insomnia is the inability to fall asleep or waking in the middle of the night and staying awake. If this problem continues for more than a month it is called chronic insomnia. Most of the cases of insomnia are related to normal day to day worries and tension or simply to caffeine consumption and is not a serious condition but it can be very frustrating and can cause lack of attention and bad temper.

Chronic insomnia is a different matter and it can interfere and disrupt a normal life. It contributes to headaches, dizziness, mental exhaustion, confusion, memory problems and emotional instability. Insomnia is not a disease but it can be a sign of a more serious disorder such as arthritis, asthma, stress, kidney, heart disease, etc.

TIP: Did you know that waking up at 1:00 to 3:00 a.m. is a sign of a liver dysfunction?

Many people turn to sleeping pills for help but this is hardly the answer to insomnia problems. These drugs cause a number of side effects including liver damage, high blood pressure and they weaken the immune system. Besides, one can very easily become dependent of them. Once they do, a higher dose is needed and when they are discontinued the use withdrawal symptoms become a major problem and insomnia resumes along with agitation and fogginess which causes people to reach for the pills again and in an even higher dose.

We are sure you will see that there is no need to put your body through pain caused by the side effects of these drugs, especially when there is a better answer in the form of natural herbs. Take a look.

We recommend

* Hops calms nerves, relieves tension and helps in cases of insomnia caused by stress, headaches and indigestion. It does not affect the early waking hours of the morning.

* A few hours before bedtime take Kava kava. It reduces stress, tension, anxiety and relaxes muscles. It helps you to fall asleep deeper and to rest more. It can be used as a sedative when taking a large dose as effectively as benzodiazepines but without the side effects.

* The most popular herb for insomnia is Valerian. It relaxes nerves and muscles, improves sleep quality and makes falling asleep easier. Great for insomnia caused by mind activity, fear, fatigue or excitement. It's as good as many barbiturates but has no side effects or addiction.

Mix the following ingredients:
    1 tsp. chamomile flowers.
    1 tsp. hops.
    1 tsp. valerian root.
    1 cup of boiling water.
Steep for 45 minutes, strain and drink 1 hour before bedtime.

Make a tea mixing the following ingredients:
    1 tbsp. of catnip leaves.
    ½ tbsp. of hops.
    1 tbsp. of chamomile flower.
    1 tbsp. of passionflower.   2 cups of boiling water.
Steep for 45 minutes, strain and drink 1 cup before bedtime.

* Catnip has sedative and tranquilizing properties. It is very good for insomnia caused by indigestion, gas, infant colic or menstrual cramps. It relaxes the body and mind during colds and flu.

* Passionflower helps if insomnia occurs from overwork, stress, pain, cough, drugs or alcohol. This is a great herb for children and infants teething, stomach pain etc. It soothes and relieves anxiety, irritability and is good for people with asthma or heart disease.

* Skullcap relieves insomnia caused by anxiety, worry or pain.

* Before going to bed, eat any of the following: bananas, milk, tuna, turkey, yogurt all of these contain tryptophan, it's been proven that they promote sleep.

* Avoid the following foods before bedtime: ham, cheese, chocolate, sausage, tomatoes, sugar.

* Do not use the bedroom for reading, watch TV, needle work etc. Go to the bedroom when you are sleepy or to for sex only.

* Jamaican dogwood is a strong pain reliever, sedative and antispasmodic. It's very helpful for muscular back pain, asthma, menstrual pain, insomnia, toothaches, and nervous conditions.

Sore throat:

A sore throat is a common and minor condition in which the back of the throat becomes irritated. Most cases (90% of them) are caused by a virus such as the one that causes colds and flu or the bacteria that cause strep infection. In cases of bacterial or viral infections antibiotics are completely ineffective and should not be taken.

Other causes of sore throat are: medication, surgery, radiation, dust, smoke, chemicals, loud talking, tooth and gum infection, allergies.

TIP: Did you know that mercury tooth filling can cause inflammation and ulceration in the mouth and throat?

In children a sore throat may be an indication of chickenpox or measles. Keep in mind other symptoms related to these diseases but remember that children show signs of a sore throat in many other illnesses.

We recommend

* Take echinacea. This herb´s antiviral and antibacterial properties speeds healing boosts the immune system.

* Horseradish is another herb that many use in the kitchen but also has excellent properties to treat sore throat and upper respiratory tract infections. It also reduces fever and expels concentrations of mucus.

* Use kava kava as a gargle for soothing and analgesic pain relief. It also helps insomnia caused by coughing and sore throat.

* Myrrh is an antiseptic and anti-inflammatory that is very powerful and excellent for a chronic sore throat. It also acts as an expectorant and decongestant and helps cure gum disease.

TIP: Store your toothbrush in grapefruit seed extract to kill

226

germs and bacteria. If you used hydrogen peroxide, wash the brush before using.

* In Europe it is common to see singers use oregano oil for its antifungal and antibacterial properties to fight respiratory allergies, laryngitis and sore throat.

* Sage is used to cure sore throat, stuffed nose, gingivitis and coughs and is a powerful antiviral, antibacterial and antifungal. Use as a gargle.

* Wild indigo is an antiviral and antibiotic for infections. It stimulates the immune system and cures a chronic sore throat.

* Mullein coats the throat with a mucus like film helping reduce a burning feeling. It clears mucus and phlegm.

* Osha is an antiviral that works great in the first stages of an infection such as colds, flu, sore throat and phlegm. It acts as an expectorant.

* Poke root relieves inflammation and infection and reduces coughing, pain and burning.

Make a gargle tonic with:
    1 cup of boiling water.
    2 tsp. sage leaves.
    salt.
mix all ingredients and let it steep for 30 minutes, drain and use as gargle when needed.

Make your own cough syrup mixing:
    1 tbsp. licorice root.
    1 tbsp. of marshmallow root.
    1 tbsp. of plantain leaves.
    1 tsp. of thyme leaf.
    4 tbsp. of honey.
    4 ounces of glycerin.
    2 drops of anise oil.
Place all herbs in a container with boiling water, let them simmer for 20 minutes, strain, add honeyand glycerin and, if desired, anise. Take 1 tbsp. as needed. Keeps in the refrigerator for several months.

TIP: Did you know that sore throat can be contracted from bacteria in toothbrushes?

Make your own sore throat tea by mixing:
  1 tsp. Canadian fleabane leaves.
  1 tsp. slippery elm bark.
  1 tsp. echinacea root.
  2 cups of boiling water.
Step for 30 minutes, strain, drink it warm up to 2 cups a day.

Make your own sore throat gargle by mixing:
  1 tbsp. of elderberry fruit juice.
  1 tbsp. of sumac extract.
  1 tsp. echinacea root extract.
Use as gargle as needed.

Heartburn:

Heartburn is a burning sensation and pain in the stomach and chest behind the breastbone. The symptoms of heartburn are the following: bloating, gas, nausea, shortness of breath and/or an acidic or sour taste in the throat and mouth.

Heartburn is caused when hydrochloric acid which is used to digest food is released up the esophagus. On its way up the acid irritates the sensitive tissues in the esophagus and throat. Usually the esophageal sphincter muscle contracts thus preventing the stomach acid from shooting up into the esophagus but if this muscle is not functioning properly the acid can slip past it and this is when heartburn symptoms start. It is called Gastroesophageal reflux disease because of the muscle malfunction but it's also known as dyspepsia, chronic heartburn or acid indigestion. If left untreated the repeated flow of acid through the esophagus can scar and produce changes in the cells lining and can cause cancer later in life.

A hiatus hernia develops when the stomach bulges up into the diaphragm. This condition can also cause heartburn. Other triggers for heartburn are alcohol drinking, smoking and eating acidic foods.

The good news is that herbs can deal with this problem very easily.

TIP: Doctors no longer recommend drinking milk to reduce heartburn. It has been proven that milk temporarily reduces the symptoms only to increase acid production by the stomach which causes more heartburn.

If you are one of those people who uses antacids, think about this next time you are about to take one. Antacids reduce nutrient absorption such as Iron and increase blood pressure. They also upset the kidneys and their relief is short.

The best solution for heartburn is the use of herbs and vegetables.

We recommend:

* Papaya chewable tablets can be purchased in health stores and they are helpful reducing heartburn.

* Drink Aloe Vera juice to heal the intestinal tract.

* Drink Chamomile tea after meals to relieve esophageal irritation.

* Doctors are using Licorice to treat heartburn and stomach and esophagus ulcers.

* Drink a large glass of water at the first sign of heartburn. If the symptoms are not too strong this will help.

* Make a juice using raw potatoes. Wash the potato very well do not peel it, just place it in the juicer, mix it with some other juice for taste and drink immediately after juicing.

* For people suffering from severe cases of heartburn or gastroesophageal disease, it is recommended that they eat lots of raw vegetables, smaller portions and chew slowly and completely before swallowing.

* Papaya seeds and pineapple aids digestion.

* Do not eat and go to bed because this increases the chance of developing heartburn. It is recommended to wait three hours after a meal before going to sleep.

* Avoid caffeine, fried foods, fats, tobacco, tomatoes, onions, and spicy foods if you suffer from heartburn.

* Remember that heartburn can be triggered by anger and stress.

* Anise improves appetite and helps digestion if taken after meals. Very helpful in heartburn, reduces infant colic, nausea, gas and cramps.

* Geranium relieves pain and acidity and accelerates healing of bleeding ulcers.

* Meadowsweet reduces stomach acidity, heartburn and nausea and aids ulcers and controls gastritis and diarrhea.

* Ginger relieves indigestion and gas and prevents and heals ulcers and reduces heartburn.

Heartburn preparation.

1 tsp. Chamomile flowers.
1 tsp. Lemon balm leaves.
1 tsp. Licorice root.
½ tsp. Slippery elm bark.
½ tsp. Fennel seeds.
½ tsp. Catnip leaves.
1 ½ cups boiling water.
1 ½ cups apple juice.
Mix herbs and cover with water. Steep for 20 minutes, strain and add juice. Drink 2 cups a day.

Gastritis

Gastritis means "inflammation of the stomach." In most cases the lining of the stomach suffers erosion and perforations, sometimes even bleeding. The most common causes of gastritis are alcohol and most pain killers. From aspirin, Advil, Motrin and Nuprin to Aleve and many others cause irritation of the gastrointestinal tract and this leads to gastritis and ulcers.

People suffering from stress are also prone to gastritis. Surgery, burns, trauma and other serious medical problems increase the chances of developing gastritis.

The way gastritis attacks the stomach walls is by disrupting the mucosa, the name given to the lining of the stomach. However, other types of gastritis produce inflammation underneath the stomach lining due to bacteria or anemia. These cases are prone to develop into ulcers.

Gastritis in most cases is painless. Common symptoms are: loss of appetite, vomiting, nausea, bloating and indigestion and some people may experience abdominal pain when eating.

We recommend:

* Eliminate dairy products from your diet until the digestive system is healed.

* Drink eight large glasses of water a day.

* Take 400 IU a day of vitamin E to reduce inflammation in the stomach.

* If your gastritis is caused by anemia, take supplemental chlorophyll two capsules three times a day and follow the recommendations under anemia.

* Licorice (DGL) helps heal the gastrointestinal tract. Chew 300 to 600 mg. 30 minutes before meals. This herb is also used to treat ulcers. Licorice is as effective as Tagamet.

* Take Artichoke if you feel abdominal pain, bloating or to relieve vomiting and nausea.

TIP: Do not use cayenne in acute cases of gastritis or ulcers.

One of the best herbs for treating gastritis is Ginger. It relieves almost all symptoms including indigestion and gas, quickly healing stomach and intestinal tissue and reduces inflammation and ulcerated linings. Ginger is an anti-inflammatory and antibacterial. It reduces nausea, stimulates digestion of fats and it's a natural antibiotic.

* Goldenseal destroys bacteria that causes gastritis, stomach inflammation and ulcers.

* Marshmallow relives nausea, indigestion, gastritis and ulcers.

* Peppermint contains volatile oils like menthol. It relieves indigestion, gastritis and stomach ulcers.

* Papaya seeds and pineapple aid digestion. It should be eaten slightly ripe. Papaya is rich in digestive enzymes.

A peptic ulcer is an area of erosion in the mucous membranes of the stomach or duodenum, the upper portion of the intestine directly below the stomach. Ulcers are in part caused (and can be worsened) by the corrosive action of the gastric acids. Gastric juices are part hydrochloric acid and part pepsin, an enzyme that helps break down food. The walls of the stomach secrete a mucus substance to protect the linings from the corrosive action of the stomach acid. However if there is too much acid or not enough mucus coating the walls of the stomach, a peptic ulcer may develop. External substances can also irritate the linings of the stomach, things like tobacco, alcohol and some drugs like Advil, Aleve, Aspirin, Motrin, etc. are also part of the ulcer causing irritants.

It's now known that a bacterium called H. pylori can also contribute to the development of ulcers. This type of bacterium is commonly found in the linings of the stomach and is the principal cause of ulcers. It has been shown that 90% of people suffering from ulcers in the duodenum and 75% of all gastric ulcers are caused by this bacteria which attacks the walls of the stomach and has been linked to gastric cancer as well.

Ulcers are very common in the bottom part of the stomach and upper part of the duodenum and men are more likely to develop ulcers than women.
The symptoms of peptic ulcers are very different from person to person. Some feel a burning pain in the stomach and others feel it in the chest. Most people feel better during meals and other feel worse eating. In any case the pain may be severe enough to cause insomnia and can be triggered by stress.

We recommend:

* It's very important to follow a diet rich in fiber and low in fats. Eat steamed green vegetables like alfalfa, broccoli and tomatoes.

TIP: Did you know that deficiency in vitamin K has been linked to ulcers? Vitamin K prevents bleeding and promotes healing. Our body produces enough of this vitamin but people with deficiency are prone to develop ulcers. Vitamin K is found in tomatoes, cheese, egg yolks, liver and in most green leafy vegetables.

* Eat small portions to avoid producing too much digestive acid but eat frequently to keep these acids from attacking the stomach linings.

* Studies have shown that cabbage juice cures ulcers in less that ten days. Prepare cabbage juice and drink one quarter a day divided in four doses (must be taken immediately after juicing). If you can't tolerate the taste or odor of cabbage there is a Chinese remedy made with dried cabbage that has been used for many years with excellent results.

* For bleeding ulcers eat organic baby food and drink brown rice water to soothe the digestive system.

* Avoid milk. Although it soothes the digestive tract and neutralizes stomach acid, it also stimulates the production of more acid further irritating the ulcerated area.

* Avoid coffee, alcohol, citrus juices, sugar and hot and spicy foods. These substances irritate the stomach and encourage the production of gastric acid.

* Take 5000 IU of vitamin A four times a day for six weeks to heal the mucus membrane.

* Take vitamin E to heal the stomach linings.

* Drink 1/4 cup of aloe vera juice a day. It's been used for centuries to relieve the symptoms of ulcers.

* Goldenseal is a natural antibiotic. Take 500 mg. of standardized extract.

* Licorice (DGL) helps heal the gastrointestinal tract. Chew 300 to 600 mg. 30 minutes before meals. This herb is also used to treat ulcers. Licorice is as effective as Tagamet.

* The homeopathic remedy carbo vegetabilis reduces the production of stomach acids and relieves the discomfort. Take 30x or 15c as needed.

* Papaya seeds and pineapple aid digestion. It should be eaten slightly ripe. Papaya is rich in digestive enzymes.

* Marshmallow relives nausea, indigestion, gastritis and ulcers.

* Stomach acid Self-Test.

If you suffer from stomach pain there is a way to find out if the problem is caused by excessive amounts of gastric acids. At the first sign of pain, swallow a tablespoon of apple cider vinegar or lemon juice. If this gets rid of the pain, you most likely have too little stomach acid but if the pain gets worse then you have too much acid and the recommendations above will help you correct the problem.

* Garlic kills bacteria and microbes and it aids the rapid healing of ulcers.

Ulcer Pain Night Reliever.

Mix the following herbs.
1 tsp. Licorice DGL extract.
1 tsp. Hops.
1 tsp. Passionflower.
1 tsp. Skullcap.
1 tsp. Valerian root.
2 cups boiling water.
Strain the herbs and let the liquid cool, Hot liquids can irritate the linings and make the symptoms worse. Drink one cup after dinner. It will reduce pain and improve sleep.

NOTE: Prescription and over the counter drugs do relieve temporarily the symptoms of ulcers but they don't treat the root of the problem. Ulcers are damaged tissue that needs to be repaired. Ulcer drugs create the illusion that the condition has been cured and this leads the person to believe that it's ok to go back to their old diets and habits. In the long term this can prove to be fatal. Many cases of stomach cancer are the result of poorly treated ulcers.

TIP: Did you know that the Cabrini Medical Center in New York has developed a method to test for the presence of ulcers using Kool-Aid ?   In the test the patient is given 2 glasses of Kool-Aid, after some time a sample of urine is tested. The sugar from the drink passes though the ulcers and it shows in the urine as undigested sugar. If the patient does not have ulcers it shows as normally broken down sugar.

Tobacco Dependency:

TIP: Did you know that every time you smoke you inhale more then 4,000 chemicals and about 50 of them cause cancer?

Every cigarette contains nicotine which we now know is very addictive and causes many problems and changes to the body. By stimulating different parts of the brain nicotine produces a feeling of pleasure in the central nervous system and also causes adrenaline production to increase, accelerates the heart rate and increases blood pressure, but that's not all, it affects the level of some hormones and the body's temperature.

All these sudden changes produced by the act of smoking are what the smoker refers to as a feeling of pleasure and is the principal fact that makes quitting smoking so hard. If we add to this the fact that nicotine is a chemical very easy to tolerate, we have in our hands one of the most powerful drugs in the world, that is completely legal and can be obtained in any convenience store.

TIP: Did you know that smoking is considered to be more addictive than cocaine?

Nicotine creates addiction very rapidly. Once hooked if the smoker stops smoking he or she will feel the symptoms of withdrawal including: frustration, anxiety, anger, lack of concentration, excess appetite, headaches, higher blood pressure and a constant craving for smoking.

Most smokers acquired the habit through peer pressure or to imitate friends or to belong to a group of people. Whatever way, smokers are usually insecure and nervous people that need the cigarette between their fingers to give them a sense of tranquility and to help them get through stressful times or awkward moments.

Like we said, smoking is an addiction that is very hard to get rid of but everyday thousands of people quit this nasty habit and so can you, especially if you follow the instructions that we are going to give you and if you use the herbs that we have found to clean nicotine from the body and reduce the cravings. YOU CAN DO IT!!! And we'll show you how.

FACT: If we take nicotine in liquid form, a drop the size of a pinhead would be enough to kill a person. Nicotine is a deadly toxin that when inhaled can cause an infinite number of diseases.

Remember this, in the United States alone, smoking kills 400,000 people a year, more than alcohol, drugs, suicide, traffic accidents and murder combined!!! It's hard to believe but is true. If we look at the rest of the world we'll find that smoking kills three million people a year. That is three million souls killing themselves and suffering a slow and painful death. But not only smokers are the affected ones, second hand smoke causes thousands of lung cancers and more then 40,000 people a year die of heart disease from second hand smoke.

Smoking causes 33% of all cancer deaths and many more diseases such as, angina, cataracts, arteriosclerosis, diarrhea, emphysema, impotence, mouth and throat cancer, heart diseases and circulatory problems.

Female smokers tend to reach menopause earlier then non smokers they are at higher risk of developing osteoporosis, cancer in the uterus and cervix. They are also less fertile and have more problems during pregnancy. They have more birth defects, miscarriages and stillborn then non smokers. Their babies are three times more likely to die of SIDS (sudden infant death syndrome) they are at risk of developing brain cancer and leukemia.

Tobacco smoke contains some dangerous chemicals including carbon monoxide, benzene, cyanide, ammonia, nitrosamines, vinyl chloride, radioactive particles and many more, in total more then 4,000 of them.

Herbs can be extraordinarily effective for quitting tobacco smoking. They reduce cravings, heal the damage done to the linings of the nose and throat, clear the lungs, and help breakdown nicotine. They also clean the blood and boost the immune system.

By using herbs the results of quitting are noticeable almost immediately. The heart rate and blood pressure go back to normal in less the 24 hours; within a week you feel that breathing is easier, oxygen levels in the blood are up 50% and carbon monoxide is down, you can smell and taste better and your chances of heart attack decrease.

We are sure that if the herbs we recommend are used in the proper way, anybody can quit smoking, no matter how long they have been addicted to it. So give yourself a chance and do it for the ones who love you and care about you.

We recommend

* Take 200 mg. twice a day of Coenzyme Q10. This is a powerful antioxidant that protects the lungs, the heart and increases oxygen to the brain.

* Take grape seed extract to repair lung damage.

* Smoking breaks down vitamin C therefore it is very important to take 5,000-20,000 mg. of vitamin C each day.

* Vitamin E is a very important antioxidant needed to repair cell damage caused by smoke.

* Vitamin A helps repair the mucus membranes which are damaged by smoking.

* For cravings, take cayenne. It desensitizes the respiratory linings to tobacco and chemical irritants. It's an antioxidant that stabilizes lung membranes preventing damage. The warm peppery taste reduces cigarette cravings.

* Ginger and Lobelia prevent nausea, helps quitting and reduces anxiety. Ginger produces perspiration which helps to shed toxins generated from smoking.

* Lobelia relieves withdrawal including irritability, hunger and poor concentration. It contains alkaloids similar to those in nicotine, occupies same brain receptor sites and exerts nicotine like effects without the damage that nicotine causes. This reduces cravings, and creates aversion.

* Oats reduce or eliminate tobacco cravings. They also, reduce the number of cigarettes desired even in those people not trying to quit.

* Plantain creates aversion to tobacco and nicotine. Helps irritability and insomnia from tobacco.

* Skullcap is a sedative and reduces anxiety and cravings.

Withdrawals Mix Tincture

½ a teaspoon of valerian rhizome tincture.
½ a teaspoon of skullcap leaves tincture.
½ a teaspoon of st. John's Wort leaves tincture.
1 teaspoon of fresh oat berries tincture.
½ a teaspoon of passionflower.
Take 5 dropperfuls a day.

* Burdock root and red clover are used to clean the blood of toxins.

* Slippery elm relieves lung congestion and coughs.

* Try fasting for a five-day period drinking fresh juices only such as carrot juice, to reduce the chance of lung cancer. Beet juice (both root and leaves) asparagus juice and apple juice can also be consumed. Remember we are talking fresh squeezed juices. This can be very powerful in getting rid of all the nicotine in your system and will reduce the cravings dramatically and it's only for five days. After that eat lots of vegetables, spinach, broccoli, sweet potatoes and whole grain (nuts). Remember also that oat, bran and wheats are needed to eliminate cravings.

* Drink lots of pure water to help these herbs and nutrients carry out the toxins and clean your blood fast.

* Yerba Santa dilates the bronchi, expels mucus, relieves wheezing and tightness.

Stress:

Stress is the body's reaction to a physical, emotional, social or mental condition imposed on the person. These changes, whether good or bad, produces tension or stress. There is no way to avoid stress completely. Injuries, weddings, meetings, childbirth, deadlines, bills to pay, even going to a party is stressful.

It's part of our daily life and is very hard to control but there are situations in life that create an extraordinary amount of stress, things like overwork, death of family or friends, surgery etc. which in turn can be damaging to our health leading to fatigue, headaches, backaches, muscle pain, stiff neck, loss of appetite, memory loss, low self esteem, lower sexual drive, changes in sleep patterns and shallow breathing. Adding all of these up results in a potential chance of becoming ill with an even more severe condition, things like high blood pressure, skin disorders, heart attacks, cancer and obesity.

We recommend

Mix 1 tsp. of valerian rhizome.
     1 tsp. of licorice root.
     1 tsp. of siberian ginseng root.
     1 tsp. of kava root.
Take one teaspoon every 3 or 4 hours.

* Take Ashwaganda. This herb comes from India, improves mental and physical performance, relaxes brain waves and reduces stress, especially in people affected by overwork, anxiety, sexual debility and fatigue.

* Ginkgo biloba improves circulation and brain activity.

* Licorice protects against damaging effects of stress, increases energy and reduces inflammation to boost the immune system.

* Siberian ginseng stimulates the immune system and gives more stamina, alertness and resistance to stress induced illness.

* Holy basil lowers stress, blood pressure and blood sugar levels. It invigorates and increases vitality.

* Ginseng reduces fatigue and regulates sleep. It controls stress from mental and physical overload and improves concentration.

* Cordyceps promotes immunity, sex drive, improves endurance, vitality and reduces exhaustion.

* Schizandra counters the effects of stress and fatigue and improves your ability to do mental and physical work.

* Kava kava relaxes the brain and body.

* St John's Wort is a good antidepressant and calms nerves.

Mix 1 tsp. of kava kava root.
    1 tsp. of hops.
    1 tsp. dried skullcap.
    1 cup of boiling water.
Let it sit for 1 hour. Strain and drink 1 tablespoon every 3 to 4 hours.

Mix 2 tsp. of valerian root.
    1 tsp. of peppermint leaves.
    1 cup. boiling water.
Steep for 45 minutes, drain and drink 1 cup per day.

* Using some or a combination of herbs we have mentioned will make you sleep better at night this is very important to achieve. Not enough sleep is one of the first symptoms that must be dealt with in order to fight stress.

* Jamaican dogwood is a strong pain reliever, sedative and antispasmodic. It's very helpful for muscular back pain, asthma, menstrual pain, insomnia, toothaches, and nervous conditions.

Things we can do to avoid stress and better our lives.

Learn to relax. Many times relaxing our body leads to relaxing of the mind.

Do not eat or drink too much caffeine. Although it gives you stamina and vitality, it also disturbs sleep patterns and makes you more nervous.

When things are not going the way you want, don't "talk down on you" the way you talk to yourself has a lot to do with the way you feel. Things like "I'll never learn this," "I can't do it" or "I hate this guy" are negative thinking and promotes stress, depression and frustration.

Take warm baths using essential oils. (Aromatherapy).

Find a hobby, something you like to do and spend time for yourself.

Take a weekend off, but don't stay home, drive to another town or to a quiet place.

Tonsillitis

Tonsillitis is an inflammation of the palatine tonsils, which are the accumulations of lymphatic tissue on the right and left sides of the upper throat. It can be caused by either viral or bacterial infection. Generally, younger children tend to get viral tonsillitis, while older children and adults tend to get bacterial tonsillitis (caused by Streptococcus bacteria). Symptoms include sore throat, difficulty swallowing, hoarseness, coughing, redness, pain and swelling. If the cases of tonsillitis are severe other symptoms may appear, like, headaches, earaches, fever, chills, nausea, vomiting, and enlarged lymph nodes in different parts of the body.

In adults this condition may be a sign of a depressed immune system resulting in the inability to fight infections and other diseases. Also improper diet (too high in refined carbohydrates and low in protein and other nutrients) may predispose one to develop tonsillitis. In some cases this condition becomes chronic, due to the repeated bouts. If left untreated tonsillitis can lead to a more sever illness called Peritonsillar abscess in which the airways become obstructed making breathing difficult. After repeated bouts the infection can spread to the neck and chest making it hard to treat. Also, scar tissue grows every time the tonsils become inflamed aggravating the symptoms and the annoyance.

A person suffering from this disease should first boost his or her immune system and then attempt to treat the condition, always as naturally as possible.

We recommend

* Take vitamin C w/ bioflavonoids 5,000 - 20,000 mg daily to fight infection and boost immune system.

* Echinacea fights infection and boosts the immune system; take as much tea as you can or take 1/2 a teaspoon twice a day of tincture.

* Pau d'arco is a natural antibiotic that improves the immune system and is also a powerful antioxidant. (see antioxidants).

* Chamomile reduces headaches, fever and pain.

Tonsillitis Pain reducer Tea.

1 tsp. elder flowers.
1 tsp. peppermint leaves.
1 tsp. yarrow.
4 cups of water.
Boil water and remove from heat, place herbs in the water and steep for 20 minutes, strain and drink 2 cups a day.

* Flaxseed oil reduces pain and inflammation and speeds recovery.

* Place a poultice made with Hot Mullein to soothe.

* Marshmallow tea coats inflamed mucous membranes. Mix 3 tablespoons of marshmallow blossoms and 3 cups of cold water, steep for 12 hours then heat and strain. Drink 2 or 3 cups a day.

Tonsillitis Gargle remedy.

2 tsp. sage.
1 tsp. alum.
4 cups of water.
Boil water and herbs and steep for 45 minutes, strain and add 5 drops of peppermint. Mix well and use it as a gargle as many times as needed.

* For a sore throat take goldenseal extract or St. John Wort extract. Six drops a day for no more than 5 days.

* Thyme reduces fever, headaches and mucus. It's very good for treating chronic respiratory problems and sore throat.

* Salt water gargles also help reduce inflammation and irritation of the throat.

* Remember that cigarette smoke irritates the mouth and throat.

Tonsillitis Steam Treatment.

Place 3 drops of lavender essential oil
       3 drops lemon essential oil.
       3 drops bergamot essential oil.

3 drops tea tree essential oil.

In 1 quart of boiling water. Place a towel over your head, lean close to the steam and inhale with your eyes closed. The fumes from the oils will relieve pain.

Wrinkles form when the skin thins and loses its elasticity. The appearance of some wrinkles is due to aging and is the most common skin problem for women. One of the first signs of wrinkles normally appear around the eye and is called " crow's feet." As time goes by the cheeks and lips are the next thing we notice. As we age, our skin becomes thinner and dryer, both factors contribute to the formation of wrinkles.

There are many factors that can contribute in the development of wrinkles some of which are: diet and nutrition, muscle tone, pollution, habitual facial expressions, chemicals, stress, improper skin care, and lifestyle habits such as smoking.

The most important factor is sun exposure which is your skin's worst enemy because it dries the skin and leads to the generation of free radicals that can damage skin cells. Research shows that 90% of what we think are signs of age are actually signs of over exposure to sunlight. Furthermore, approximately 70% of sun damage comes from everyday activities such as driving and walking to and from your car.

The ultraviolet-A rays that cause this enormous damage are present all day long in all seasons. These ultraviolet-A rays wear away the elasticity of the skin, causing wrinkling. The worst part is that the effects of the sun are cumulative, although they may not be noticeable for many years.

TIP:Did you know that natural beauty products are not always as advertised?

Manufacturers say that their products contain natural ingredients but the reality is that they contain tiny amounts compared to the artificial substances used. You find out by looking at the label of the product. The ingredients are listed in descending order, starting with the greatest amount contained. For example, a product may be labeled as rosemary, but the label shows only chemicals and artificial substances and not a drop of pure rosemary.

We recommend:

* Eat a balanced diet including fruits, vegetables, whole grain foods, seeds, nuts and legumes.

* Drink plenty of fluids every day. This help to keep the skin hydrated and flush away toxins.

* Obtain fatty acids from cold pressed vegetable oils.

* Avoid alcohol, caffeine and cigarettes. They dry the skin and encourage the development of wrinkles. Also the smoking habit uses the lips' muscles hundreds of times a day which contributes to wrinkling.

* Always protect your skin from the sun by applying a sunscreen with a sun protection factor (SPF) of at least 15 to all exposed areas of the skin.

* Avoid alcohol-based products. Use hazel or an herbal, floral water instead.

* Avoid using harsh soaps or solid cleansing creams. Use natural oils such as avocado oil to remove dirt and makeup.

* Do not apply heavy oils around the eye area before going to bed. Because it might cause the eye to be puffy in the morning.

* Take Vitamin E to protect against free radicals that can damage the skin and contribute to aging and wrinkles.

* Take Vitamin C to promote the formation of collagen, a protein that gives the skin flexibility. It also fights free radicals and strengthens the capillaries that feed the skin.

* Take Silica. It is important for skin strength and elasticity and also, stimulates collagen formation.

* Take Vitamin A. It is necessary for healing and the construction of new skin tissue.

* Take Vitamin B complex + Vitamin B12. They are anti stress and anti aging vitamins.

* Take primrose or black currant seed oil. They are good healers for dermatitis, acne and others skin disorders.

* Use a collagen cream because it is very good for dry skin.

* Use elastin cream to help smooth existing wrinkles and prevent the appearance of new ones.

* To alleviate puffy eyes, peel a cucumber, cool it and place it in the eye area for 10 minutes. Repeat if necessary.

* To cleanse the pores, rub mush tomatoes over your face, then rinse.

* To protect your skin from free radical damage, add a few drops of green tea extract to your lotions or astringents.

* To moisture your skin, mash together grapes and honey, enough to make a paste, apply over your face as a mask. Leave it for 30 minutes then rinse away.

* To remove dead cells and improve skin texture, rub a small handful of dry short grain rice against your face for a couple of minutes.

* To soften and nourish the skin, mash half an avocado and apply over the face. Leave it on until it dries, then rinse with warm water.

Home Remedies For Allergies

An allergy is a hypersensitive reaction to a normally harmless substance. There are a variety of substances, termed allergens, that may trouble a sensitive individual. Common allergens include pollen, animal dander, house dust, feathers, mites, chemicals, and a variety of foods. Some allergies primarily cause respiratory symptoms; others can cause such diverse symptoms as headache, fatigue, fever, diarrhea, stomachache, and vomiting. This entry addresses respiratory allergies, both chronic and seasonal (for a discussion of allergic reactions caused by foods. Home remedies for allergies can help reduce and treat allergies symptoms.

If you have allergies, you may suffer from a stuffy and/or runny nose, sneezing, itchy skin and eyes, and/or red, watery eyes. Needless to say, it can be very uncomfortable. These symptoms occur because, in the presence of an allergen, the immune system releases chemicals called histamines to fight what it perceives as an invader. Home remedies for allergies can treat all of the above mentioned symptoms.

Histamines cause a string of reactions, including the swelling and congestion of nasal passages and increased mucus production. This is essentially a hypersensitive, or overactive, response by the body to an external stimulus. You will not suffer any of these side effect using this home remedies for allergies.

Whether allergies are seasonal or chronic depends on the particular allergen or allergens involved. Seasonal allergies tend to be caused by pollen. Ongoing or chronic allergies are usually caused by factors that are present in the environment year-round, such as animal dander, dust, or feathers. Chronic allergic rhinitis is a persistent inflammation of the mucous membrane lining the nasal passages that is caused by an allergic reaction. It is characterized by a stuffy, runny nose, frequent sneezing, and a tendency to breathe through the mouth. The eyes may be red and watery. Headache, itchiness, nosebleeds, and fatigue may be secondary complications. Dark circles under the eyes (called "allergic shiners"), along with a puffy look to the face, are frequently seen.

Home remedies for Allergies - Diet

Home remedies for allergies #1: ■ Drink lots of water to thin secretions and ease expectoration.

Home remedies for allergies #2: ■ If you have respiratory allergies, you may be allergic to certain foods. In addition to dairy products and wheat, common culprits include eggs, chocolate, nuts, seafood, and citrus fruits and juices. Try eliminating one of these foods for two weeks and watch for an improvement. Use an elimination or rotation diet to discover and work with food allergies.

Home remedies for allergies #3: Try eliminating dairy foods from your diet. Dairy foods can thicken mucus and stimulate an increase in mucus production. If your allergies are seasonal, it may also be helpful to avoid whole wheat during the allergy season; many allergy sufferers are sensitive to wheat.

Home remedies for allergies #4: Cut out cooked fats and oils. When your body is under any type of stress, including the stress of an allergic reaction, the digestive system is not as strong as usual, and fats—which are difficult to digest at the best of times—can put a strain on the digestive system. Also, undigested fats contribute to mucus production and foster a toxic internal environment.

Home remedies for Allergies - Supplements

Home remedies for allergies #5: Calcium and magnesium are important nutrients for the allergy sufferer. They help to relax an overreactive nervous system. While symptoms are acute, take a supplement containing 750 to 1,000 milligrams of calcium and 500 milligrams of magnesium twice a day. Then take the same dosage once a day for two months.

Home remedies for allergies #6: Allergies are often related to the transformation and transportation of foods in the digestive system. Taking a digestive-enzyme supplement will enhance the assimilation and utilization of nutrients. Take a full-spectrum digestive-enzyme supplement providing 5,000 international units of lipase, 2,500 international units of amylase, and 300 international units of protease, plus 500 to 1,000 milligrams of pancreatin immediately after each meal.

Home remedies for allergies #7: Methylsulfonylmethane (MSM) is a good source of sulfur, a trace mineral that may help to reduce the severity of the allergic response. Take 500 milligrams three or four times daily, with meals.

Home remedies for allergies #8: Selenium is an antioxidant and works synergistically with vitamin E. Take 50 to 100 micrograms twice a day during the allergy season.

Home remedies for allergies #9: Vitamin C has anti-inflammatory properties. During acute flare-ups, take 1,000 milligrams five times a day for four to five days. Follow this with 1,000 milligrams three times a day for three weeks; then take 1,000 milligrams a day for two months. Some people with allergies find mineral ascorbate vitamin C or esterified vitamin C (Ester-C) easier to tolerate than simple ascorbic acid.

Home remedies for Allergies - Herbs

Home remedies for allergies #10: If your nasal mucus is green or yellow, you may have an infection on top of allergies. Take one dose of an echinacea and goldenseal combination formula supplying 250 to 500 milligrams of echinacea and 150 to 300 milligrams of goldenseal two to three times daily for five to seven days to help resolve the infection.

Home remedies for allergies #11: Nettle can be very helpful for drying out the sinuses. It can be highly effective for chronic allergies. Take 150 to 500 milligrams two or three times daily, as needed, for two weeks.

Home remedies for allergies #12: Turmeric is an East Indian herb with natural anti-inflammatory properties. It is an excellent remedy for those who suffer from fatigue coupled with allergies. Take 500 milligrams three times daily.

Home Remedies For Headache

Virtually everyone gets a headache at one time or another. An estimated 17.6 percent of women and 6 percent of men in the United States experience headaches on more than an occasional basis, and some 20 million regularly experience cluster and migraine headaches. Home remedies are the best way to treat a headache because they are as common—and as difficult to cure—as the common cold and flu. Common causes of headache include stress; tension; anxiety; allergies; constipation; coffee consumption; eyestrain; hunger; sinus pressure; muscle tension; hormonal imbalances; temporomandibular joint (TMJ) syndrome; trauma to the head; nutritional deficiencies; the use of alcohol, drugs, or tobacco; fever; and exposure to irritants such as pollution, perfume, or after-shave lotions. Migraines result from a disturbance in the blood circulation in the head. (See MIGRAINE)

Headache experts estimate that about 90 percent of all headaches are tension headaches and 6 percent are migraines. Tension headaches, as the name implies, are caused by muscular tension. Another type of headache is the cluster headache. These are severe, recurring headaches that strike about 1 million Americans, and are widely considered to be the most painful type of headache.

Using home remedies for headaches is a great way to get rid of the pain without using drugs. Headaches can also be a sign of an underlying health problem. People who suffer from frequent headaches may be reacting to certain foods and food additives, such as wheat, chocolate, monosodium glutamate (MSG), sulfites (used in restaurants on salad bars), sugar, hot dogs, luncheon meats, dairy products, nuts, citric acid, fermented foods (cheeses, sour cream, yogurt), alcohol, vinegar, and/or marinated foods. Other possibilities to consider are anemia, boWel problems, brain disorders such as tumors, bruxism (tooth-grinding), hypertension (high blood pressure), hypoglycemia (low blood sugar), sinusitis, spinal misalignment, toxic overdoses of vitamin A, vitamin B deficiency, and diseases of the eye, nose, and throat. Dehydration also can cause headaches—often accompanied by a feeling of being flushed, a warm face, and a sense of heaviness in the head.

Unless otherwise specified, the dosages recommended here are for adults. For a child between the ages of twelve and seventeen, reduce the dose to three-quarters the recommended amount. For a child between six and twelve, use one-half the recommended dose, and for a child under the age of six, use one-quarter the recommended amount.

Home remedies for Headaches

Home remedies for headaches #1: Coenzyme Q10 plus
Coenzyme A Improves tissue oxygenation. Take 30 mg twice daily.

Home remedies for headaches #2: Calcium and magnesium are Minerals that help to alleviate muscular tension. Use chelated forms.
Deficiency may be a cause of migraines. Relaxes muscles and blood vessels. Take 1,000 mg daily.

Home remedies for headaches #3: Glucosamine sulfate is a natural alternative to aspirin and other nonsteroidal anti- inflammatory drugs (NSAIDs).

Home remedies for headaches #4: Cayenne thins the blood, which reduces pain and allows beneficial blood flow.

Home remedies for headaches #5: Chamomile relaxes muscles and soothes tension.

Home remedies for headaches #6: Ginkgo biloba extract improves circulation to the brain, and may be helpful for certain types of headache.

Home remedies for headaches #7: Guarana can alleviate cluster headaches.

Home remedies for headaches #8: Use a homeopathic remedy suitable for the particular headache symptoms you are experiencing. Belladonna helps with sudden, severe pain that is worse on the right side, of the body. Natrum muriaticum is recommended for tension headaches and periodic headaches. Sanguinaria is good for pain that is sharp and splitting. Arsenicum album, kali bichrornium, Mecurius solubilis, and Pulsatilla all encourage drainage of the sinuses.

Home Remedies For Anxiety

Anxiety is the second most common psychological problem, yet remains undiagnosed 75% of the time. In our anxious age, doubts and fears can manifest as simple worries, free-floating anxiety, phobias (agoraphobia, social phobias, etc.), panic disorders and obsessive-compulsive tendencies. The latter may affect as many as 7 million Americans. Home remedies for anxiety offer the best approacho to complement the traditional treatment.

Physical aspects of anxiety include stomach upsets, colitis, migraines, palpitations, hypertension and sweating. Anxiety after trauma, post traumatic stress syndrome (PTSD), is also increasingly common. Underlying, contributing factors are low blood sugar, food allergy, nutrient deficiency (fatty acids, B complex, etc.) and imbalances of the thyroid, ovaries or adrenals. Home remedies for anxiety can help you get this nutrient in.

Many of the herbs that help anxiety work on the same brain receptor sites as drugs like Valium, Xanax and Halcion. Herbs however, tend to be gentler, safer and non-addictive. They have relaxant properties but also nourish and strengthen the nervous system. There are hundreds of home remedies for anxiety and nervous disorders.

Home remedies for Anxiety

Home remedies for Anxiety #1: California Poppy**—Eschscholtzia californica
· A tension-relieving, sedative, anti-anxiety and antispasmodic herb.
· Helps sleeplessness, quells headache and muscular spasm from stress.
· Gentle, non-addictive action that is safe for children and the elderly.

Home remedies for Anxiety #2: Chamomile***—Matricaria recutita
· Tranquilizing effects, with action similar to drugs, i.e. Halcion, Valium.
· Reduces effects of stress-induced chemicals in the brain, while promoting healthy adrenal hormones (e.g. cortisol). Relieves pain and spasms.
· Aids digestion, cramping and back pain. Promotes restful sleep.

Home remedies for Anxiety #3: Hops**—Humulus lupulus
· Calms nerves, eases anxiety, restlessness and tension. For headaches from stress, insomnia / sleep loss, indigestion or effects of alcohol.
· Its sedative properties are not appropriate for use during depression.

Home remedies for Anxiety #4: Kava Kava***—Piper methysticum
· Reduces anxiety, fear, tension; alleviates stress from many emotional, interpersonal and career factors. Improves performance; no grogginess.
· Relaxes muscles, relieves pain, insomnia and promotes restful sleep.
· Compares favorably to tranquilizers and benzodiazepines for anxiety.

Home remedies for Anxiety #5: Lemon Balrn*—Melissa officinalis
· Relaxing and tonic herb, reduces anxiety, restlessness and nervousness.
· Helps with panic disorder, palpitations, racing heart, overactive thyroid.

· For digestive upset from stress or anxiety; nausea, indigestion, colic.
· Anti-depressant. Good in synergistic combination with other herbs.

Home remedies for Anxiety #6: Linden**—Tilia europaea
· Reduces tension, promotes relaxation; mild mood-elevating qualities.
· Protects against illness due to stress, anxiety and overactive adrenal glands, including high blood pressure, palpitations, gastric ulcers.

Home remedies for Anxiety #7: Mothervvort**—Leonarus cardiaca
· A relaxing, tonic herb and mild sedative that gently relieves tension, anxiety when feeling under pressure. A heart, uterine and thyroid tonic.
· Relieves symptoms like a racing heart, shallow breathing.

Home remedies for Anxiety #8: Passionflower* *—Passiflora incarnata
· Sedative herb that relieves anxiety, tension, spasms, pains, neuralgia.
· Promotes restful, refreshed sleep; induces relaxation, mild euphoria.
· Gentle action, suitable for nervousness in children and the elderly.

Home remedies for Anxiety #9: Skullcap***—Scutellaria laterifolia
· Relaxes, yet tones and renews the nervous system. Calms oversensitivity.
· Helps hysteria, depression and exhaustion, eases stress during PMS.
· Pain reliever and antispasmodic, decreases restlessness, nervousness.

Home remedies for Anxiety #10: St. John's Wort***--Hypericum perfoliatum
· Effective long-term action for anxiety and tension, as well as irritability and depression. Also for mood changes during menopause and for pain syndromes, including fibromyalgia, arthritis and neuralgia.

Home remedies for Anxiety #11: Valerian* * *—Valeriana officinalis
· Sedative and muscle relaxant; for anxiety, stress, muscle tension and pain, nervous cramps, restlessness, insomnia, overwork or overstudy.
· For easing off drug dependency (both medical and recreational drugs).
· For after effects of chronic flu. Improves poor concentration.

Home remedies for Anxiety #12: Vervain**—Verbena officinalis
· Relaxing nervine; reduces tension, strengthens the nervous system.
· Reduces anxiety due to stress, PMS or menopause, calms hysteria.
· Useful for lingering depression after a cold or flu. Tones the liver.

Home remedies for Anxiety #13: Wild Lettuce*--Lactuca virosa
· Gentle tranquilizer, calming an overactive, excitable nervous system.
· Very suitable for anxious children or adolescents. Helps with insomnia.
· General pain reliever and antispasmodic, especially for irritable coughs.

Home remedies for Anxiety #14: Wood Betony**—Stachys officinalis
· Sedative action, relieves tension, anxiety and nervous exhaustion.
· Calms an overactive, edgy state. Relieves headaches and neuralgic pain.
· Strengthens neurological function and improves memory, clarity.

Home Remedies For Attention Deficit Disorder

Attention deficit disorder and hyperactivity are the epidemic of our age, but current treatment is woefully inadequate. While our society wages an ongoing "war on drugs," millions of children are hooked on "speed" in the form of Ritalin and amphetamines. Apart from serious and permanent side effects, these do not remotely address underlying causes and can in no way be regarded as a cure. In the other hand home remedies for ADD and ADHD are a great natural alternative if you want your child to remain drug free.

Diagnoses such as learning disability, hyperactivity and poor impulse control are usually attributed to a brain chemistry imbalance. A better term might be "toxic brain syndrome," since the overriding factor is a constant bombardment of the child's nervous system with pesticides, mercury, lead, food additives, artificial sweeteners, vaccines, antibiotics and allergenic foods. Each one of these factors has been shown to significantly and profoundly impact developing brain cells and combine together with devastating effects. Home remedies for ADD and ADHD are free of chemicals and side effects.

A full-scale assault on these problems requires a homeopathic, herbal and nutritional program to undo the developmental and biological damage caused by chronic exposure to toxins. Home remedies for ADD and ADHD have the short- term gain of relaxing and calming, while improving brain function and neurotransmitter production. In the long run, nervine and adaptogenic plants can protect, detoxify and heal the nervous system—all without the significant toxicity or side effects of drugs. See also Anxiety - Fatigue - Insomnia - Depressions - Memory -Stress to treat ADD and ADHD with home remedies.

Home remedies for Attention deficit disorder

Home remedies Attention deficit disorder #1: Bacopa**—Brahmi/Bacopa monnieri
· Calming and sedative. Improves attention deficit disorder; important for hyperactivity.
· Improves intellectual capacity, acuity, clarity of thought, concentration.
· Improves memory, especially in the elderly; shortens learning time.

Home remedies Attention deficit disorder #2: California Poppy***—Eschscholtzia californica
· A gentle sedative that relieves psychological and emotional disturbances in kids. Soothes and balances an overactive nervous system.
· Reduces attention deficit disorder and tension in overactive states, decreases spasms.
· Effective for difficulty in falling asleep or frequent, regular waking.

Home remedies Attention deficit disorder #3: Catnip*—Nepeta cataria
· Relieves attention deficit disorder, restlessness, tension, stress and hyperactivity.
· A mild relaxant that promotes restful sleep. Helps diarrhea, headache, colic or stomach ache due to stress. Balances mood swings or hysteria.

Home remedies Attention deficit disorder #4: Ginkgo**—Ginkgo biloba
· Improves focus, memory, cognition, knowledge retention, perception.
· Increases neurotransmitters, boosts the brain's ability to use oxygen.
· Increases circulation to brain; high in nutritive antioxidants that protect the brain and nervous system from damage by various toxins.

Home remedies Attention deficit disorder #5: Grape Seed Extract***—Vitis vinifera
· Contains bioflavonoids with the most potent antioxidant effects known.
· Able to cross the blood brain barrier and directly protect the brain against a wide variety of toxins and damaging free radicals.
· Improves brain blood flow, strengthens brain capillaries.

Home remedies Attention deficit disorder #6: Hops**—Humulus lupulus
· Indicated for nervous tension, excitability, restlessness and irritability.
· Excellent for insomnia, taken orally or as a hops and lavender pillow.
· Calms and improves the mood, but should be avoided in depression.
· Strengthens and stimulates digestion, relieves intestinal discomfort.

Home remedies Attention deficit disorder #7: Kava Kava**—Piper methysticum
· Valuable in attention deficit disorder; relieves attention deficit disorder without any cog-
nitive or mental impairment. Reduces insomnia, tension and stress.
· Produces a sense of tranquility and softens angry or violent feelings.
· Significantly improves mood, tension level and sleep patterns.

Home remedies Attention deficit disorder #8: Lemon Balm**—Melissa officinalis
· A gentle, safe and calming children's herb for depression and attention deficit disorder.
· Relaxes the nervous system; eases agitation while soothing digestion.

Home remedies Attention deficit disorder #9: Oats***—Avena sativa
· Nervous system nutritive and tonic for mental stress, nervousness, overwork, exhaustion, weakness. Improves mental concentration, focus.
· Eases stress, tension, depression, insomnia—but improves clarity.
· Excellent for transitioning and weaning off neurological medications.

Home remedies Attention deficit disorder #10: Skullcap**—Scutellaria laterifolia
· Helps attention deficit disorder, restlessness, crying spells, irritability and nervousness.
· A useful daytime sedative, with no mental impairment or drowsiness.
· Nervine action relieves frequent headaches, relaxes muscular spasms.

Home remedies Attention deficit disorder #11: St. John's Wort***—Hypericum perforatum
· An herb of choice for attention deficit or hyperactive children.
· Calms an agitated nervous system, yet safe for long-term usage.

· Regulates mood and attention, relieves feelings of sadness, apathy, low self-esteem, isolation, anger, guilt, shame. Good for nervous exhaustion.

Home remedies Attention deficit disorder #12: Valerian***—Valeriana officinalis
· Relaxing and sedating, reduces restlessness, nervousness, improves sleep; should be taken for 2-4 weeks to improve mood and sleep.
· Shows improvements in learning skills, with less aggressive behavior.

Why use home remedies attention deficit disorder?

The prescription medication methylphenidate (Ritalin) has become the most commonly prescribed medication to ease hyperactivity. Researchers are discovering, however, that this medication has many potentially serious, longterm side effects including decreased appetite, weight loss, insomnia, slowed growth, increased heart rate, increased blood pressure, a period of increased irritability and intolerance at the onset of use, and the possibility of developing Parkinson's disease. Increasing adverse reports have been released in recent years, warning parents of the possible side effects of Ritalin—with some reports even comparing it to cocaine.

Other prescription medications often prescribed include detroamphetamine (Dexadrine, a stimulant that produces calming effects equivalent to Ritalin), pemoline (Cylert, a stimulant that has been restricted by the FDA to use as a secondary medication because it can cause liver failure), methamphetamine (Desoxyn), amphetamine-dextroamphetamine combination (Adderall), and tricyclic antidepressants (if depression is suspected). For periods of extreme anger and aggression, a tranquilizer called thiordazine (Mellaril) may be prescribed, but it should be used only as a last resort. Various side effects, some of them seri ous, have been reported with all of these medications.

Due to the many potentially harmful side effects of the medications available for ADD/AD-HD sufferers, a growing number of parents and health professionals are turning to all or a combination of the following as a way to reduce, and even possibly eliminate the symptoms of ADD/ ADHD: alteration of diet; vitamin and mineral supplementation; herbal remedies; counseling; and the love and support of family, teachers, and friends. Many believe that medicating the problem is merely masking the symptoms without getting to the root of the problem.

Home Remedies For Yeast Infection

Systemic infection with candida and other strains of
yeast is epidemic today and is an underlying factor in many chronic conditions (e.g.
migraines, colitis, obesity, fibromyalgia, chronic fatigue, sinusitis, PMS). This is a
result of immune failure and contributes to immunity's progressive weakening. Home
remedies for yeast infection can also be used in combination with other remedies for the
above mention symptoms.

Other contributing causes include antibiotics, which destroy protective intestinal
bacteria, and a variety of immune-damaging factors and environmental toxins. Sugar
and carbohydrate excess, or estrogen imbalance (hormone therapy` pill, PMS),
sweetens the tissues, creating a yeast breeding ground. Food allergies and a toxic
digestive system (dysbiosis) complete the picture. Home remedies for yeast infection
can reverse the imbalance and return it to normal levels.

Antifungal herbs must be used and alternated for some time. An integral part of
treatment is yeast die-off or Herxheimer reaction, which can produce fatigue,
headaches, digestive upset and so on. The side effects can be minimized by starting with
low dosages, increasing gradually, and helping detoxification. A low-carb, high-protein
diet, digestive enzymes, liver detoxification and immune-strengthening herbs are
essential. Check below a list of home remedies for yeast infections. See also **Candida**

Home remedies for Yeast Infection

Home remedies for Yeast Infection #1: Black Walnut**—Juglans nigra
· Unripe, green hulls contain juglone, an effective antifungal agent.
· Assists with systemic candida, athlete's foot and ring worm infections.
· Also inhibits other fungi, cryptococcus, salmonella, staph, E. coli.

Home remedies for Yeast Infection #2: Cat's Claw* * *—Una de gato/Uncaria
tormentosa
· Has antimicrobial effects for fungi, viruses, bacteria, parasites.
· Important intestinal cleanser for dysbiosis, leaky gut, diverticulitis, colitis, Crohn's.
Anti-aging, anti-inflammatory, immune strengthening.

Home remedies for Yeast Infection #3: Celandine*--Chelidonium majus
· Treats candida effectively; powerful liver detox fier and hepatic strength-
ener; helps in removal of candida metabolites from the bloodstream.

Home remedies for Yeast Infection #4: Garlic***—Allium sativa
· Contains several antifungal ingredients; rapidly destroys yeast.
· Stimulates immune function. Highly antiseptic, effective in infections, and is
beneficial for long-term use against chronic candida syndromes.

Home remedies for Yeast Infection #5: Goldenseal***—Hydrastis canadensis
· Strong antifungal effects, while healing intestinal mucus linings.
· Strengthens and detoxifies the liver; immune and white cell stimulant.

Home remedies for Yeast Infection #6: Yeast infection Tinture:
1 ounce tincture of black walnut husk (fresh)
1/2 ounce each tinctures lavender flowers, valerian root, pau d'arco.
10 drops tea tree oil.
Mix all the ingredients and shake well before each use. Take 2 to 3 dropperfuls a day.

Home Remedies For Fatigue Syndrome

Fatigue is the most common presenting complaint in doctor's offices, and can be part of scores of serious medical conditions, as much as from overwork or lack of sleep. Underlying causes need to be identified, and natural medicine recognizes many less obvious contributing factors. These include chronic intestinal dysbiosis, liver overload, adrenal exhaustion, hidden infections (yeast, viral or parasitic) and food allergies. Typical short-term solutions such as caffeine, tobacco, sugar and other stimulants are ultimately debilitating for the hormonal and nervous system. That is why home remedies for fatigue syndrome are the best long term option to compliment your treatment.

Herbal medicines should be directed toward the underlying causes, but for simple fatigue, tonic and adaptogenic herbs can be relied upon. These have the ability to increase vitality and well-being, balancing and improving the function of the body's major control systems—immune, hormonal, cardiovascular and nervous. Thus they are particularly suitable for the effects of prolonged stress, both physical and psychological. This class of botanical medicines can help compensate for and overcome the effects of overwork, depression, prolonged illness and convalescence after illness. In this list of home remedies for fatigue syndrome you will find the whole spectrum of benefits.

Optimal effects occur when tonics are taken long term (i.e. one to six months). They are best taken in chronic illness, rather than acutely and are typically used in a cycle of 3 weeks on and one week off. See also Immune Weakness - Liver Conditions - Stress.

Home Remedies for Fatigue Syndrome

Home Remedies for Fatigue #1: Alfalfa**—Medicago sativa
· Improves appetite, digestion; produces mental clarity and well-being.
· Increases stamina and strength, augments ability to respond to stress.
· For convalescence after long illness, extreme stress. Reduces toxicity.
· High in phytoestrogens, stimulates the body's hormone production.
· Note that alfalfa sprouts and especially seeds are potentially toxic.

Home Remedies for Fatigue #2: Astragalus*** —Milk Vetch/Astragalus membranaceous
· For general weakness, fatigue, loss of appetite, shortness of breath.
· Adaptogenic herb that stimulates immune function, improves stamina.
· Anti-inflammatory, antiviral, antibacterial effects; good for flu, cold.
· Strengthens people with cancer, after radiation or chemotherapy.

Home Remedies for Fatigue #3: Cordyceps**—Cordyceps sinensis
· Builds strength, endurance, stamina and immunity. Reduces fatigue, promotes lung and kidney function. Increases blood flow to brain, heart.
· Increases male potency, female vitality. Improves appetite and sleep.

Home Remedies for Fatigue #4: Ginseng***—Panax Ginseng
· Strengthens adrenals, improves vitality and ability to handles stress.

· Improves physical and mental performance, stamina; enhances mood.
· Increases visual and motor coordination, increases work capacity.
· Antioxidant, inhibits formation of free radicals, stimulates immunity.

Home Remedies for Fatigue #5: Gotu Kola***—Centella asiatica
· Improves brain function, memory. Anti-stress, anti-anxiety, relaxant.
· Strengthens body's connective tissue and blood vessels, heals wounds.
· Tonic and rejuvenator, improves fertility, has anti-inflammatory effects.

Home Remedies for Fatigue #6: Licorice**—Glycyrrhiza glabra
· Provides steroid-like factors for the the body's own production of adrenaline, cortisol; thus boosts adrenal function and adaptation to stress.
· Antiviral and immune-enhancing herb, valuable for weakened states.

Home Remedies for Fatigue #7: Maitake**—Grifola frondosa
· Immune-stimulating effects; increases activity of immune cells (killer cells, etc.), as well as immune-modulating chemicals (interleukin 2).
· D-fraction has shown positive results in Epstein-Barr and chronic fatigue; inhibits virus production, protects cells from attack by toxins.

Home Remedies for Fatigue #8: Oats***—Avena sativa
· Exhaustion from work, study, illness, drugs, alcohol, sexual excess.
· Nutritive effect on the brain, rather than temporary stimulatory effect.
· Greatly sharpens mental acuity, focus, memory before an exam etc..
· Eases heart palpitations, effective for insomnia due to overfatigue.

Home Remedies for Fatigue #9: Schisandra***—Schisandra chinensis
· Improves adrenal and nervous system capacity. Counteracts effects of stimulants, coffee. Improves liver function and protects it from toxins.
· Increases work and efficiency level, improves mood, memory and sleep.
· Re-regulates immune system, helps skin problems, aphrodisiac effects.

Home Remedies for Fatigue #10: Siberian Ginseng***—Eleutherococcus senticosus
· Adaptogenic herb, excellent for exhaustion, fatigue, immune weakness.
· For effects of long stress (physical, emotional, mental) or after illness.
· Increases mental alertness, work output and athletic performance.
· Enhances adrenals, increases immunity and protects against toxins.

Home Remedies for Fatigue #11: St. John's Wort*—Hypericum perforatum
· Inhibits viral activity and replication of herpes virus and Epstein-Barr.
· Relieves depression that is a cause or effect of fatigue; improves sleep.

Home Remedies for Fatigue #12: Yerba Mate*—Ilex paraguariensis
· Stimulates like caffeine, but without causing nervousness; calms, balances the nervous system. Improves sleep and mood, reduces allergy.
· Antioxidant, increases oxygen to the heart and brain.

Home Remedies For Candida

The human body is normally host to a great variety of bacteria and fungi that play neutral or even helpful roles in normal bodily functions. A candida occurs when one of the these organisms, the yeast Candida albicans, grows out of control. The resulting overgrowth is known as candidiasis. C. albicans only becomes a problem when the "good" bacteria that normally keep it in check, such as Lactobacillus acidophilus, become weakened. Candida infection may take the form of athlete's foot and jock itch. Use home remedies for candida is a great alternative.

Systemic candidiasis is an overgrowth of candida throughout the body. In the most severe cases, candida can travel throughout the body, causing a type of blood poisoning called candida septicemia.

Candidiasis affects both women and men. It is rarely transmitted sexually. It is most common in babies (an infected mother may pass it on to her newborn) and people with compromised immune systems. As it proliferates, the fungus releases toxins that further weaken the immune system. Home remedies for candida can also be used with remedies for the immune system.

Because candidiasis can affect many areas of the body at once, it can cause a variety of disorders and symptoms. In the mouth, C. albicans can produce thrush, or white plaques in the mouth and throat. In women, it is one of the sources of vaginitis, which produces itching, burning, and a sticky white or yellow discharge. Overgrowth of yeast may result in weak nails; skin infections, marked by redness, inflammation, and itching; or digestive upsets causing abdominal pain, constipation, diarrhea, heartburn, rectal irritation, and colitis. candidas may develop in the urethra or sinuses. Other symptoms can include fatigue, memory loss, mood swings, muscle and joint pain, nagging cough and congestion, and numbness or tingling in the fingers and toes. Home remedies for candida can help with many of these symptoms.

Additional symptoms can include diaper rash, kidney and bladder infections, canker sores, headaches, and depression. candida may also be implicated in some cases of impotence and prostatitis.
The growth of C. albicans is spurred by several factors. Broad-spectrum antibiotics can kill off the good bacteria that keep the yeast under control. Home remedies for candida can be used with regular antibiotics.

Taking corticosteroid drugs has been linked to C. albicans overgrowth. C. albicans is a sugar-loving organism, so candidiasis can be aggravated by eating too much sugar, or by the high blood-sugar levels associated with diabetes. And yeast can overgrow if the immune system does not function as it should, especially in people with HIV infection or AIDS and other diseases that affect the immune system. An imbalance in PH levels in the body is also a likely cause. C. albicans overgrowth is also associated with chronic fatigue syndrome, and with chronic skin or vaginal irritation. Home remedies for candida reduce irritation and discomfort.

Conventional medicine uses various antifungal agents. Except for barberry and related herbs, which should not be used for more than two weeks at a time, it may be necessary to take herbs for as long as six months to control yeast overgrowth.

Home remedies for candida

Home remedies for Candida #1: Take Lactobacillus and bifidus probiotic supplements daily. These friendly bacteria grow to form a protective lining over the digestive tract that keeps yeast colonies from forming. Be sure to check expiration dates on the package. For vaginal infections, place the probiotic capsules in the vagina before going to bed every other night for two weeks.

Home remedies for Candida #2: Take 1,000 to 2,000 milligrams of caprylic acid daily with meals. This naturally occurring fatty acid is an effective antifungal for the treatment of candida. Since caprylic acid is readily absorbed by the intestines, it is necessary to take a timed-release or enteric-coated form so that the supplement is released gradually throughout the entire digestive tract.

Home remedies for Candida #1: Avoid refined sugar, honey, maple syrup, and fruit juices. Also avoid chewing gums flavored with xylitol, which may aggravate thrush. ❏Avoid antibiotics, steroids, and birth control pills unless medically directed to take them.

Home remedies for Candida #3: Several different antifungal agents are used to treat yeast
infections. Topical creams include butoconazole (Femstat 3) and miconazole (Monistat), some of which are now available without prescription. Nystatin (Mycolog, Mycostatin, Nilstat) is relatively safe because it is not absorbed from the gastrointestinal tract. Stronger agents include fluconazole (Diflucan), itraconazole (Sporanox), and ketoconazole (Nizoral). Use of ketoconazole should be avoided, if possible, since this drug can be toxic to the liver. If ketoconazole is called for, its use should be supervised by an infectious disease specialist.

Home remedies for Candida #4: If you take the prescription blood-thinner warfarin (Coumadin), you should consult your doctor before using over-the-counter vaginal miconazole products. Miconazole is an antifungal drug found in some creams and suppositories used to treat vaginal candida. Bleeding or bruising may occur if warfarin and vaginal miconazole are used together.

Home remedies for Candida #5: In otherwise healthy people, high sugar consumption has very little effect on the growth of yeast. Only when the balance of yeast and other naturally occurring bacteria is upset by antibiotic treatment or injury to the immune system does yeast overgrowth become a problem.

Home remedies for Candida #6: While yeast overgrowth in the mucous membranes lining the gastrointestinal tract, throat, nose, urethra, and vagina are relatively common, candidas of the blood and inner organs are extremely rare. The effects of candida on the endocrine, immune, and nervous systems are caused by changes in absorption of nutrients rather than by the candida itself.

Home remedies for Candida #7: If a breast-fed baby develops oral thrush or a nursing mother develops a thrush infection of the nipples, both the mother and the baby should be treated to eradicate the infection, even if only one of them seems to be affected.

Home Remedies For High Blood Pressure

Whether blood pressure is high, low, or normal depends on several factors: the output from the heart, the resistance to blood flow of the blood vessels, the volume of blood, and blood distribution to the various organs. All of these factors in turn can be affected by the activities of the nervous system and certain hormones. Home remedies for high blood pressure can treat many symptoms to help regulate blood pressure naturally.

If blood pressure is elevated, the heart must work harder to pump an adequate amount of blood to all the tissues of the body. Ultimately, the condition often leads to kidney failure, heart failure, and stroke. In addition, high blood pressure is often associated with coronary heart disease, arteriosclerosis, kidney disorders, obesity, diabetes, hyperthyroidism, and adrenal tumors. There are many great home remedies for high blood pressure in this site.

The list of circulatory disorders is almost endless and includes heart disease, strokes, hypertension, and atherosclerosis, to name a few. These and other circulatory conditions are the number-one cause of death in this country, killing nearly one million Americans every year. You could be a victim of this silent killer, make it a habbit to use home remedies for high blood pressure to lower the risks.

As we age, our body's ability to keep a proper equilibrium between blood clotting and blood liquefaction begins to go awry. On the one hand, blood must clot if we are to keep from bleeding to death, yet, on the other hand, it must be free flowing and liquid in order to travel easily through the body's blood vessels. The older we get, the "stickier" our blood gets, and our blood's ability to flow diminishes. When this occurs, the stage is set for blood clots, clogged arteries, strokes, and heart attacks.

Warning signs associated with advanced hypertension may include headaches, sweating, rapid pulse, shortness of breath, dizziness, and visual disturbances.

Home remedies for high blood pressure

Home Remedies for High Blood Pressure #1:
Use cayenne (capsicum), chamomile, fennel, hawthorn berries, parsley, and rosemary for high blood pressure.
Caution: Do not use chamomile on an ongoing basis, as ragweed allergy may result. Avoid it completely if you are allergic to ragweed.

Home Remedies for High Blood Pressure #2: Hops and valerian root are good for calming the nerves.

Home Remedies for High Blood Pressure #3: Drink 3 cups of suma tea daily.

Home Remedies for High Blood Pressure #4: Avoid the herbs ephedra (ma huang) and licorice, as these herbs can elevate blood pressure.

Home Remedies for High Blood Pressure #5: Follow a strict salt-free diet. This is essential for lowering blood pressure. Lowering your salt intake is not enough; eliminate all salt from your diet. Read labels carefully and avoid those food products that have "salt," "soda," "sodium," or the symbol "Na" on the label. Some foods and food additives that should be avoided on this diet include monosodium glutamate (Accent, MSG); baking soda; canned vegetables (unless marked sodium- or salt-free); commercially prepared foods; over-the-counter medications that contain ibuprofen (such as Advil or Nuprin); diet soft drinks; foods with mold inhibitors, preservatives, and/or sugar substitutes; meat tenderizers; softened water; and soy sauce.

Home Remedies for High Blood Pressure #6: Eat a high-fiber diet and take supplemental fiber. Oat bran is a good source of fiber.
Note: Always take supplemental fiber separately from other supplements and medications.

Home Remedies for High Blood Pressure #7: Eat plenty of fruits and vegetables, such as apples, asparagus, bananas, broccoli, cabbage, cantaloupe, eggplant, garlic, grapefruit, green leafy vegetables, melons, peas, prunes, raisins, squash, and sweet potatoes.

Home Remedies for High Blood Pressure #8: Include fresh "live" juices in the diet. The following juices are healthful: beet, carrot, celery, currant, cranberry, citrus fruit, parsley, spinach, and watermelon.

Home Remedies for High Blood Pressure #9: Eat grains like brown rice, buckwheat, millet, and oats.

Home Remedies for High Blood Pressure #10: Drink steam-distilled water only

Home Remedies for High Blood Pressure #11: Take 2 tablespoons of flaxseed oil daily

CIRCULATORY TEA #1
- teaspoon burdock root
1 teaApoon goldenAeal root
- teaApoon cayenne
2 teaspoons slippery elm bark
2 AliceA ginger root
3 cups boiling water
Combine the above herbs in a nonmetallic container, and pour the boiling water over them. Steep for 3o minutes, cool, and strain. Take up to one cup a day, two tablespoons at a time.

CIRCULATORY TEA #2
teaspoons black cohoAh root
4 teaspoons ginkgo biloba leaves cups boiling water
Combine the above herbs in a nonmetallic container, and pour the boiling water over

them. Soak for 3o minutes, cool, and strain. Take two to three tablespoons at a time, up to six times a day.

Home Remedies For Nausea and Vomiting

Nausea is an unpleasant feeling that you are about to vomit. It is often accompanied by excess salivation and sometimes stomach cramping. A number of diseases and conditions can cause nausea, including food poisoning (and other bacterial infections), viral infections, overeating or overdrinking, gallstones, pancreatitis, and cancer. It can also occur because of motion sickness, headache, or pregnancy. There are some very powerful home remedies for nausea and vomiting.

Sometimes unpleasant smells or tastes, and even emotional anxiety, can bring on nausea.
In addition to those herbs listed below, other beneficial herbs to relieve nausea include bayberry, bee balm, chaparral, horehound, and Oregon grape. These are great herbs to make home remedies for nausea and vomiting.

Home remedies for nausea and vomiting

Home Remedies for nausea and vomiting #1:
NAUSEA TEA #1
1 teaspoon grated ginger root 1 teaApoon yerba mama root
1 teaspoon peppermint leaves
2 cups boiling water
Combine the above herbs in a nonmetallic container and cover with the boiling water; steep for 3o minutes; cool and strain. Take as needed, a tablespoon at a time up to two cups a day.

Home Remedies for nausea and vomiting #2: NAUSEA TEA #2
1 tcaspoon catnip leaves
1 teaspoon chamomile flowers cup boiling water
Combine the above ingredients in a nonmetallic container and cover with the boiling water; steep for zo to 3o minutes; cool and strain. Take as needed.

Home Remedies for nausea and vomiting #3: Cayenne***—Capsicum frutescens
· Anti-inflammatory; relieves nausea, vomiting, gas, indigestion.
· Promotes digestion, warms the stomach and stimulates appetite.
· Do not use in acute stages of inflammatory gastritis or stomach ulcer.

Home Remedies for nausea and vomiting #4: Chamomile***—Matricaria recutita
· Tranquilizing effects with action similar to drugs like Halcion, Valium.
· Reduces effects of stress-induced chemicals in the brain, while promot-

ing healthy adrenal hormones (e.g. cortisol). Relieves pain, spasms.
· Also aids digestion, cramping, back pain. Promotes restful sleep.

Home Remedies for nausea and vomiting #5: Cinnamon*—Cinnamomum zeylandicum
· Relieves nausea, vomiting. Treats gastroenteritis, stomach flu, diarrhea.
· Antibacterial, antiviral and antifungal; expels gas, reduces spasms.
· Warming, astringent and stimulating to the digestion, reduces mucus.

Home Remedies for nausea and vomiting #6: Cloves*—Eugenia caryophyllata
· Relieves nausea, prevents vomiting. Reduces gastrointestinal spasms.
· Expels gas, bloating; antibacterial and antiviral, eliminates parasites.
· A few drops of the oil or infusion may be taken for quick nausea relief.

Home Remedies For Hives *Urticaria*

Hives, called urticaria by the medical profession, is a skin condition that is characterized by sudden outbreaks of red, itchy welts on the skin. Any area of the body may be affected. The welts may vary in appearance, from tiny, goosebump-like spots to rashes that cover significant areas of the body. Hives usually go away within a few hours to two days, but in rare cases they become chronic and may last for six weeks or more. Home remedies for hives urticaria can greatly reduce the time of the outbrake.

Many cases of hives are brought on as allergic reactions and coincide with the release of histamine in the body. The release of histamine into the skin produces an inflammatory reaction, with itching, swelling, and redness. Hives can cause significant discomfort, but it does not cause injury or damage to any vital organs. However, home remedies for hives urticaria help also improve the immune system.

The skin is the largest organ of the body. It is an important part of the excretory system. The skin acts in conjunction with other systems in the body to remove toxins and waste. Hives can be a natural reaction to the presence of a foreign substance in the body. However, an offending substance need not enter the body to trigger an outbreak of hives. Home remedies for hives urticaria can treat the skin naturally.

Merely coming into contact with various substances, such as pesticides, soaps, shampoos, hair sprays, residues from laundry products or dry cleaning chemicals on clothing, or any other of a vast array of other seemingly innocuous household items can unleash a maddening attack of hives.
The severity of a hives outbreak can vary from case to case as well as from person to person. Some people can break out in hives if they merely touch a certain type of plant or bush; others may develop hives only with considerable exposure, such as overconsumption of a certain food. Chemicals are a major cause of hives for many people; anything from perfumes to household cleaners can trigger a reaction, as can nervous conditions, stress, certain foods, and alcohol.

Viruses also can cause hives. Hepatitis B and Epstein- Barr virus, the virus that causes infectious mononucleosis, are the two most common culprits. Some bacterial infections likewise can cause outbreaks of hives, both chronic and acute. An association between Candida albicans and chronic hives has been established in several clinical studies over the past twenty years.

Home remedies for Hives *Urticaria*

Home Remedies for Hives *Urticaria* #1:
Aloe**—Aloe vera
· Applied topically, reduces inflammation, provides protective coating.
· Cooling to the tissues, relieves itching, redness, stinging and pain.
· Internally, stimulates immunity and elimination of inflammatory toxins.

Home Remedies for Hives _Urticaria_ #2: Bromelain***—Pineapple/Ananas comosus
· More effective anti-inflammatory than most drugs, decreases the allergic response, alleviating hives, skin irritations. Accelerates healing.
· Non-toxic in large internal doses; may be applied directly to the hives.

Home Remedies for Hives _Urticaria_ #3: Burdock**—Arctium lappa
· A liver and blood detoxifier, diuretic, digestive stimulant; assists in clearance of cellular and lymphatic debris, reduces tissue swelling.
· Purifies skin problems such as hives, acne, boils, eczema and psoriasis
· Stimulates the immune system; antibacterial, antiviral, antifungal.

Home Remedies for Hives _Urticaria_ #4:
Chinese Skullcap**—Scutellaria baicalensis
· Contains potent flavonoids that are anti-allergic and anti-inflammatory.
· Stabilizes body during increased immune stress or allergen overload.
· Cools conditions of "damp heat" such as hives, fever, infections.

Home Remedies for Hives _Urticaria_ #5: Curcurnin***—Turmeric/Curcuma longa
· Stimulates the body's natural anti-inflammatory corticosteroids.
· Very effective natural antihistamine and antioxidant for hives and a variety of inflammatory skin ailments. Protects liver against toxins.

Home Remedies for Hives _Urticaria_ #6: Echinacea* * *—Echinacea angustifolia
· Anti-inflammatory; reduces sensitivity to allergens, stings or bites.
· Encourages blood and lymph drainage, modulates and balances a hyper-reactive immune system. antiviral and antibacterial effects.

Home Remedies for Hives _Urticaria_ #7: Ginger* * *—Zingiber officinale
· Rapidly quells the onset of hives, itching or other allergic responses.
· A potent anti-inflammatory and antihistamine, improves skin circulation, relieves swelling and carries away inflammatory waste products.

Home Remedies for Hives _Urticaria_ #8: Goldenseal/Coptis/Oregon Grape**—
Berberis spp
· Soothing herbs for swelling, itching; ideal for hives and skin disorders such as boils, sores, abscesses and fluid-filled or pustular eruptions.
· Tonic and detoxifying to the liver, gall bladder, stomach and intestines.

Home Remedies for Hives _Urticaria_ #9:
Green Tea***—Camellia sinensis
· Strong antihistamine, reducing hives and other allergic inflammations.
· High in antioxidant polyphenols and flavonoids that protects against oxidative, toxic damage to the tissues. Enhances the immune system.

Home Remedies for Hives _Urticaria_ #10: Licorice**—Glycyrrhiza glabra
· Antihistamine and anti-inflammatory, increases levels of cortisone.
· Immune stimulating, improves stress response, antiviral activity.
· DGL form is not effective for allergy. Also use locally as a tea or lotion.

Home Remedies for Hives *Urticaria* **#11:** Nettles***—Urtica dioica
· Freeze-dried form provides fast-acting antihistamine, symptom relief.
· Anti-inflammatory and astringent to relieve swelling or edema of hives.
· Detoxifying and diuretic, encourages excretion of inflammatory wastes.

Home Remedies for Hives *Urticaria* **#12:** Quercetin***—Quercetin
· A non-toxic, potent antihistamine bioflavonoid, decreases inflamma-
tion of allergic skin and hay fever conditions. Strengthens capillaries
· May be taken acutely during hive outbreak or as a preventive measure.

Home Remedies for Hives *Urticaria* **#13:** Schisandra**—Schisandra chinensis
· Chinese herb that alleviates hives, eczema and swollen tissues.
· A tonic for the adrenals, increases ability to deal with chemical stress.
· Improves sluggish or deficient liver and protects it from various toxins.

Home Remedies for Hives *Urticaria* **#14:** Yarrow***—Achillea millefolium
· Pain-relieving astringent, antiseptic and anti-inflammatory action.
· Take internally or apply directly to hives to quell inflammation and pain
associated with swollen tissues. Detoxifies tissues of cellular waste.

Cuts and scrapes are breaks in the skin that are inevitable in the course of life. They can be painful, interfering with movement and activities. Cuts can bleed profusely, especially if they are on the head, face, hands, mouth, or feet, where there are many blood vessels close to the surface of the skin. They can become infected, especially if they are on the face, fingers, and hands, which are not normally covered with clothing. These are very common injuries and home remedies for cuts can cam very handy.

Cuts can leave scars. Special attention should be given to those on the face and lips so that there will be no noticeable lasting skin defect. Cuts on the lips often require stitches to heal properly. Stitches may be required to close larger wounds elsewhere to effect minimal scarring. The more severe the cut, the more underlying tissues may be involved and the longer it may take to heal. Home remedies for cuts can speed up healing.

You can treat minor cuts and scrapes at home with basic first aid and home remedies for cuts. However, if the pain from a cut is severe, if bleeding cannot be stopped, if redness and tenderness develop around the wounds, if a cut is deep or long, or if it involves your lips, consult your physician or go to the emergency room of the nearest hospital immediately.

Home remedies for Cuts

Home remedies for Cuts #1: The following vitamin and mineral supplements are recommended to aid in rapid healing:

Home remedies for Cuts #2: Beta-carotene. Take 25,000 international units a day.

Home remedies for Cuts #3: Vitamin B6 (pyridoxine). Take 50 milligrams a day

Home remedies for Cuts #4: Vitamin C. Take 3,000 to 5,000 milligrams a day.

Home remedies for Cuts #5: Vitamin E. Take 400 international units a day

Home remedies for Cuts #6: Zinc. Take 50 to 100 milligrams a day.

Home remedies for Cuts #7: If the cut is superficial, after cleaning you can cover the cut with a mixture of zinc oxide cream and vitamin-E oil.

Home remedies for Cuts #8: Calendula gel or ointment stimulates fast healing at the skin's surface, and is a good choice for a nice clean wound. It is been endorsed by Commission E, the body of experts that advises the German government about herbs, for reducing inflammation and promoting wound healing.

Home remedies for Cuts #9: Clove oil is high in eugenol, a compound that is both an antiseptic and a painkiller. You can sprinkle powdered cloves on a cut to prevent infection.

Home remedies for Cuts #11: Comfrey roots and leaves contain allantoin, which stimulates cell division and speeds wound healing and scar formation. You can take some fresh leaves and rub them directly on your cuts and scrapes. You can also find commercial cream formulations of comfrey in many health food stores. Do not to take comfrey internally, however.

Home remedies for Cuts #12: Echinacea is also Commission E-approved as a topical treatment for superficial cuts. This herb has powerful immune-stimulating properties. You can also drink a cup of echinacea tea three to four times a day to strengthen your immune system to speed healing.

Home remedies for Cuts #13: Goldenseal contains several antiseptic compounds. You can apply a poultice of crushed goldenseal root to any minor cuts.

Home remedies for Cuts #14: Yarrow is excellent for stopping bleeding. Just sprinkle powdered yarrow extract onto the cut. Yarrow leaves and flowers have been used since ancient Roman times for their blood-clotting, anti-inflammatory, and pain-relieving qualities.

Home remedies for Cuts #15: There are a number of herbal first-aid creams available, including calendula in echinacea-and-comfrey combinations; calendula blended with white sage, elder flower, and chickweed; and calendula mixed with goldenseal, propolis, and myrrh to make topical botanical antiseptics.

Home Remedies For Hair loss in Women

You could lose at least 100 of your 100,000 scalp hairs each day So you shouldn't be alarmed if this is the case with you. Usually, the lost hair is replaced by a new hair from the same hair follicle, located just below the scalp's surface. Luckly we have some great home remedies for hair los in women to speed up growth.

Women also lose more hair as they age. Many experience a generalized thinning of the hair or a "widened part" in the center of the scalp after menopause. This is called female pattern baldness.

As with male pattern baldness, hormonal changes and genetic predisposition are to blame. Although they do not usually lose as much hair as men do, women are also constantly searching for a cure for this distressing problem. All in all, more than two-thirds of all men and women have some type of hair loss or thinning during their lifetime.

Premature hair loss or thinning can also be due to a wide variety of other causes. Most women lose quite a bit of hair in the two to three months after they deliver a baby, and this can continue for up to six months. One and a half to three months after severe stress, operation, infection, or high fever, a person may also lose a lot of hair. Likewise, two to three months after crash dieting with insufficient protein intake, hair may come out in handfuls.

Many prescription drugs can cause reversible hair loss. Cancer patients treated with certain chemotherapeutic drugs may lose up to 90 percent of their scalp hair, but it eventually returns after their treatment is finished. Birth control pills that contain high levels of progestin also can cause hair loss.

Other possible causes of hair loss include trauma; syphilis; tumors; thyroid disease; connective tissue diseases; bacterial, fungal, or herpes infections of the scalp; improper hair care with tight hairstyles, overbrushing, or overuse of dyes and permanents; and, in women, too-high levels of male hormones.

Many different nutrient deficiencies result in hair loss, including deficiencies of vitamins A, B6, B12, folic acid, biotin, vitamin C, copper, iron, and zinc. Hair loss can be a sign of vitamin A toxicity as well as deficiency. Vitamins B6, B12, folic acid, copper, and iron are necessary for the normal formation of red blood cells that supply oxygen to the hair shaft.

Copper also functions in the formation of hair pigmentation, so copper deficiency can also cause color changes in the hair. With vitamin-C deficiency, the hair splits and breaks easily, resulting in dry, kinky, tangled hair. Silica also is important for hair growth and strength. Vitamin E is also necessary for good scalp and hair follicle health.

There is also an immune problem known as alopecia areata, in which the hair suddenly comes out in totally smooth, round patches. This condition can cause a lot of pyschological stress. A person with alopecia areata can also lose hair from his or her eyelashes, eyebrows, beard, and the other hairy areas of the body.

Because a full head of hair is associated with virility, youth, and attractiveness, hair loss and thinning can have a huge negative psychological impact on a person. If you start losing more hair than normal, a dermatologist will try to identify the cause by taking a complete history doing blood tests, and examining your hair visually, under the microscope, with hair analysis, and, perhaps, with a scalp biopsy.

Home remedies for hair loss in women #1:
A high-potency multivitamin and multimineral daily.
· Beta-carotene. Take 25,000 international units daily.
· Vitamin-B complex. Take a supplement containing 100 milligrams of most of the major B vitamins. Also take an additional 50 milligrams of biotin daily.
· Vitamin C. Take 1,000 milligrams twice a day.
· Vitamin E. Take 400 international units daily, with 100 micrograms of selenium to aid its absorption.
· Iron. Take 50 milligrams daily.
· Zinc. Take 50 milligrams daily, with food and with 2 milligrams of copper.
· Silica. Take 250 milligrams twice a day.
· Free-form amino acid complex. Take 2 grams (2,000 milligrams) three times a day, before or after meals.

Home remedies for hair loss in women #2: In addition to correcting any vitamin deficiencies, women whose hair loss is due to physical trauma, crash diets, or heavy menstrual periods can benefit from supplementation with a high-potency multivitamin and 50 milligrams of iron, together with 1,000 milligrams of vitamin C to boost iron absorption.

Home remedies for hair loss in women #3: Thinning hair can be a sign of poor nutrient absorption, which in turn can be due to an insufficient supply of stomach acid or bacterial overgrowth in the stomach. Taking one tablet of hydrochloric acid (HC1) and one digestive enzyme capsule after starting each meal, plus 1/2 teaspoon of powdered acidophilus dissolved in 2 ounces of water twice a day between meals, can aid in nutrient absorption.
· Inositol with choline has been found to stimulate hair regrowth in some people with nonscarring alopecia. Take 200 milligrams twice a day.

Home remedies for hair loss in women #4:
Saw palmetto is the first choice of many herbalists for male pattern bald ness. Saw palmetto blocks the formation of dihydrotestosterone, a hormone thought to kill off hair follicles and lead to androgenic alopecia. Take 160 milligrams twice a day.
DS Some people have had success using aloe. It is suggested that you apply the gel to the scalp every night before bed, and also take 2 tablespoons of aloe juice orally each day.

Home remedies for hair loss in women #5: Arnica can be applied to the scalp twice a day in the form of a cream, ointment, or hair rinse made from arnica tincture diluted with warm water. Arnica increases local blood circulation, and may thereby help promote hair growth.

Home remedies for hair loss in women #6: Arnica can be applied to the scalp twice a day in the form of a cream, ointment, or hair rinse made from arnica tincture diluted with warm water. Arnica increases local blood circulation, and may thereby help promote hair growth.

Home remedies for hair loss in women #7: Jojoba oil may help with hair loss when applied to the scalp.

Home remedies for hair loss in women #8: Emu oil, or kalaya oil, is recommended as a moisturizer and hair-root stimulant to promote hair growth.

Home remedies for hair loss in women #9: Licorice also contains a chemical that prevents testosterone from being changed to dihydrotestosterone. You can add licorice tincture or extract to your favorite shampoo.

Home remedies for hair loss in women #10: Rosemary has long been believed to keep hair healthy and lush. Add one part rosemary oil to two parts almond oil and massage the mixture into your scalp for twenty minutes a day.

Home remedies for hair loss in women #11: Sage has been believed for centuries to help prevent hair loss. Like licorice, sage extract can be added to your favorite shampoo. Or you can use double-strength sage tea daily as a hair rinse to encourage hair growth.

Home remedies for hair loss in women #12: Safflower is considered to be a good vasodilator. Massage your scalp with safflower oil for twenty minutes a day to increase local blood flow and stimulate hair growth.Jojoba oil may help with hair loss when applied to the scalp.

Canker Sores are painful small, craterlike ulcers. They are gray-based with red rims. They usually develop on the insides of the cheeks, the inner lips, and the loose parts of the gums, mouth, and lips. Less commonly, they can affect the esophagus and rest of the gastrointestinal tract. Home remedies for canker sores can help reduce pain and speed up healing.

There is usually a burning and tingling sensation starting twenty-four hours before the ulcers actually form, and it is most helpful to start treatment as soon as this is felt. Canker sores can be so painful that they interfere with speaking, eating, and nutrition. The best alternative for healing canker sores is to use home remedies.

If they are less than one centimeter (about one-half inch) in diameter, they are called minor aphthous ulcers. These usually heal by themselves within a week or two. If they are greater than 3 centimeters in diameter, they are classified as major aphthous ulcers, and it often takes six weeks for them to finally heal. When they do, they leave scars. Both small and large ulcers often return, either singly or in crops.

Canker sores are the most common disorder to affect the oral mucous membranes, with between 20 and 50 percent of Americans affected. Women are more likely to be affected than men, usually starting in their twenties or thirties. Some people seem to have an inherited tendency to form canker sores. These people should always use home remedies to treat canker sores to avoid constant use of hash drugs.

Canker sores may be infectious, resulting from a local bacterial or viral infection. They commonly have one or more triggers, including food allergies, acidic mouth conditions, minor injury to the tissues of the mouth, smoking, vitamin deficiencies, stress, extreme heat, fever, and premenstrual and postmenopausal hormonal changes. People with poorly functioning immune systems are also very susceptible to canker sores. Home remedies for canker sores can be use in combitation with remedies for low immune system.

Home remedies for Canker Sores

Home remedies for canker sores #1: · Canker sores may be due to a deficiency of vitamin B12, folic acid, zinc, the amino acid lysine, or iron, so these nutrients may need to be supplemented aggressively. The following supplements are recommended for people with canker sores:

Home remedies for canker sores #2: · Vitamin B12. Take 1,000 micrograms daily. Also take a vitamin-B complex with 100 milligrams of most of the major B vitamins three times a day, with meals.

Home remedies for canker sores #3: · Vitamin C with bioflavonoids. Take 1,000 milligrams three times a day, with meals.

Home remedies for canker sores #4: · Zinc. Take 50 to 100 milligrams a day.

Home remedies for canker sores #5: · Iron. Take 15 milligrams a day.

Home remedies for canker sores #6: · Folic acid. Take 400 milligrams twice a day.

Home remedies for canker sores #7: · L-Lysine. Take 4 grams (4,000 milligrams) daily for the first four days, then cut back to 500 milligrams three times a day. Take this supplement on an empty stomach.

Home remedies for canker sores #8: Supplementation with acidophilus powder or capsules to restore the healthy balance of bacteria in the mucous membranes of the mouth is often helpful.

Home remedies for canker sores #9: · Applying the oil from one vitamin-E capsule directly to the sores helps to clear the lesions more quickly.

Home remedies for canker sores #10: Aloe vera juice, available by the gallon, swished around in your mouth three times a day like a mouthwash, often yields good results. Aloe contains salicylates, which are anti-inflammatory and relieve pain, and it also has mild antibacterial properties.

Home remedies for canker sores #11: Chlorophyll is a blood detoxifier. Chlorophyll tablets are sometimes chewed for the treatment of canker sores.

Home remedies for canker sores #12: A soothing antiseptic mouth rinse can be made of 1/2 teaspoon of goldenseal powder and 1/4 teaspoon salt dissolved in 1 cup of warm water. Use this as a mouth rinse four times a day. Goldenseal helps reduce inflammation of mucous membranes, and has also been shown to have antibacterial properties.

A boil or furuncle is a bacterial infection with pus that develops around a hair follicle. Boils are very contagious and potentially serious if the infection spreads. A boil starts out as a tender, red, hot, tense bump and develops a yellowish point within 2 to 4 days. Boils are very painful, especially if they occur in skin that cannot move freely. The boil can burst open, discharging pus but relieving some of the pain. There are many home remedies for boils that can reduce the symptoms.

Unfortunately, boils heal with scarring.

Boils usually occur in areas that are hairy or that are exposed to lots of movement and friction. These include areas under the belt and on the neck, face, scalp, underarms, and buttocks. Boils can become chronic and come back time and again in the same areas. Our home remedies for boils reduce the risk of developing chronic boils.

The most common bacteria found in boils is Staphylococcus aureus (staph bacteria). They may be caused by other types of bacteria, however, depending on the location of the boil and the individual's immune function. In rare cases, boils may be a sign of an underlying immune problem or other disease. People with diabetes, alcoholism, cancer, or HIV/AIDS, and those on chemotherapy are especially susceptible to developing boils. Please use these home remedies for boils.

Home remedies for boils

Home remedies for boils #1:
· Vitamin A. Take 25,000 international units daily for two weeks.

Home remedies for boils #1:
· Beta-carotene. Take 25,000 international units daily for two weeks.

Home remedies for boils #2:
· B-complex vitamins. Take a balanced B-complex supplement daily

Home remedies for boils #3:
· Vitamin C with bioflavonoids. Take 3,000 milligrams daily.

Home remedies for boils #4:
· Zinc. Take 50 milligrams daily for two weeks.

Home remedies for boils #5:
• Astralagus tea helps to enhance immunity. Drink eight glasses a day.

Home remedies for boils #6: Calendula ointment can to applied to the skin overlying an unbroken boil to decrease inflammation and act as an antiseptic.
is Garlic is a natural antibiotic and immune-system booster. It can be taken in capsule form.

Home remedies for boils #7: · Goldenseal-root powder can be mixed with enough boiling water to
make a paste and used as a topical poultice to draw out the boil.

Home remedies for boils #8: A mixture of 25 grams (2,500 milligrams) of powdered slippery elm, 3 drops of eucalyptus oil, and just enough boiling water to form a thick paste can be applied to the boil. Leave it on until the paste cools, then make a fresh batch and reapply it. Repeat this until the pus is discharged from the boil. Marshmallow leaf or figwort can also be made into a poultice to draw out pus.

Home remedies for boils #9: Tea tree oil can be applied externally to a boil as an antiseptic against bacteria and fungi. The pure oil will probably irritate inflamed skin, but a mixture of a few drops in a couple of tablespoons of any vegetable oil should not cause a problem. Do not take tea tree oil internally.

Home remedies for boils #10: · A tea made from two parts wild indigo to one part each of echinacea, pasque flower, and poke root can be drunk three times a day to speed healing. The tea can also be applied externally to a boil to limit infection.

Unpleasant body odor, or bromhidrosis, is most frequently due to excessive perspiration from the eccrine or apocrine sweat glands. This in turn causes an overgrowth of bacteria on the skin. The bacteria break down the top layer of skin cells and the sweat, forming chemicals that produce the unpleasant smell. Home remedies for body odor can control bacteria.

Apocrine bromhidrosis rarely occurs before puberty, since the apocrine sweat glands virtually do not function before then. As most apocrine sweat glands are located in the armpits, this is the smelliest area. Home remedies for body odor can help you make your own natural deodorant.

People in groups that tend to have larger numbers of apocrine sweat glands, such as people of African ancestry, are affected to a greater extent than those who tend to have fewer apocrine sweat glands, such as older adults and people of Asian descent. Poor hygiene, of course, is another reason unpleasant smells come off the body. Diet can also be a factor.

Sweat containing high levels of garlic, curry, or other spices also has a repellent odor. Taking certain medications can cause bad body odor, too.

Excessive eccrine sweating of the feet, most common in young men, is another common cause of bad body odor. Bromhidrosis from the feet occurs when the thick, warm, sodden skin becomes a breeding ground for numerous bacteria. Eccrine bromhidrosis can also occur in areas where skin contacts skin, especially between the thighs. This can be made worse by obesity and diabetes. Using home remedies for body odor can help reduce foot odor.

Other, more serious causes of offensive body odor include nutrient deficiencies, such as zinc deficiency; underlying medical problems such as genetic metabolic disorders, liver disease, or diabetes; and gastrointestinal problems such as parasites or chronic constipation. You should seek your physician's expertise to screen for these problems if excessive sweating, poor hygiene, or a spicy diet are not factors in causing the unpleasant body odor.

Home remedies for body odor

Home Remedies for body odor #1:
NUTRITIONAL SUPPLEMENTS FOR BODY ODOR:
· The following supplements have been found to be helpful for body odor:
· Vitamin A. Take 25,000 international units daily for two weeks.
· Vitamin-B complex. Take a supplement containing 100 milligrams of each of the major B vitamins daily Also take an additional 50 milligrams of vitamin B6 (pyridoxine) daily and 50 milligrams of vitamin B1 (thiamine) twice a day while the problem exists, then cut back to 20 milligrams every other day for three weeks.

· Vitamin C. Take 3,000 milligrams daily
· Zinc. Take 50 milligrams daily.

Home Remedies for body odor #2:

HERBAL TREATMENT FOR BODY ODOR:

Alfalfa tablets contain a lot of chlorophyll, which has a deodorizing effect.

· Chlorophyll, available in soft gel capsules and chewable tablets, helps reduce embarrassing body odors.

· Parsley also is a good source of chlorophyll. Munching on several sprigs of parsley a day can help with body odor.

Home Remedies for body odor #3:

NATURAL DEODORANT FOR BODY ODOR:

· Make an herbal spray deodorant by combining 5 drops each of sage, coriander, and lavender essential oils with 2 ounces of distilled witch hazel. Shake before each use.

Addiction is a complex mix of physical and psychological causes, but for many people, alcohol is a form of self-medication, related to low levels of brain chemicals, such as serotonin, dopamine and noradrenalin. Alcohol is the oldest intoxicant and addictive, in use for over 10,000 years. Alcohol directly damages the liver, esophagus, stomach, intestines and colon, and greatly increases the risk of various cancers. It is a special risk to pregnant woman, who should avoid it completely, since irreversible fetal alcohol syndrome can occur at low doses. Alcohol is also involved with an estimated 60% of all violent crimes. Despite these negatives, only 20% of alcoholics can stop successfully.

Herbal medicines offer a valuable resource for the effects of, and addiction to, alcohol. Initially, there are herbs to detoxify and lessen cravings, while reducing the symptoms of withdrawal. Acorn tincture (Quercus glandis) or angelica can be used in all cases to create a powerful aversion to alcohol. Other plant medicines help repair the damage done, including liver herbs like milk thistle. Adaptogenic and tonic herbs can correct biochemical and neurological imbalances that contribute to drinking, by doing such things such as increasing the manufacture of neurotransmitters like serotonin.

Others herbs can help underlying anxiety or depression.

Home remedies for Alcohol Detox

Home remedies for Alcohol Detox #1: Acorn***—Quercus robur glandium
· Diminishes alcoholic craving, antidotes its effects, such as enlarged spleen and liver. Diarrhea may appear during treatment as a curative effect.
· Available as a homeopathic liquid under the name Ouercus glandis.

Home remedies for Alcohol Detox #2: Angelica**—Angelica atropurpurea
· Reduces craving or creates dislike for alcohol; use 5 drops, 3 times daily.
· A warming circulatory tonic that relieves gas, bloating, colic, headache.
· Helps with enlarged spleen; anti-inflammatory and antispasmodic.

Home remedies for Alcohol Detox #3: Calanatts*—Acorus calamus
· Reduces the craving for alcohol; restorative for brain, nervous system.
· Relieves gas, cramps, distention. Improves appetite, helps exhaustion.

Home remedies for Alcohol Detox #4: Cayenne***—Capsicum frutescens
· Helps stop morning vomiting and gnawing stomach, reduces intense cravings for alcohol and promotes appetite; use in single drop doses.
· Reduces irritability, anxiety and tremor and induces calm sleep.
· Delirium tremens, chills, exhaustion can often be speedily relieved.

Home remedies for Alcohol Detox #5: Celandine***—Chelidonium majus
· Specific for liver problems from alcohol; extreme sensitivity to, and bad effects from, drinking. Liver healer and detoxifier, even for cirrhosis.

· Calms emotions (i.e. anger, depression) during withdrawal or cravings.
· For general sluggishness, difficulty concentrating and mental dullness.

Home remedies for Alcohol Detox #6: Hops**—Humulus lupulus
· Sedative that relieves anxiety-related withdrawal symptoms; aids DTs.
· Helps irritability and restlessness, promotes healthy digestion.
· Relieves insomnia, frequent wakings; not suitable during depression.

Home remedies for Alcohol Detox #7: Khella**—Ammi visnaga
· Ayurvedic herb that alleviates the acute and chronic effects of alcohol.
· Powerful antispasmodic and pain remedy. Used for asthma, angina.

Home remedies for Alcohol Detox #8: Kudzu***—Pueraria lobata
· Traditional use in China to sober a drunk person and for various side effects of alcohol (hangover, thirst, gastric bleeding, loss of appetite).
· Recent research shows it can dramatically reduce craving for alcohol.

Home remedies for Alcohol Detox #9: Milk Thistle**—Silybum marianum
· Protects against damage to the liver by alcohol, drugs and toxins.
· Powerfully regenerates damaged liver tissue; essential for cirrhosis.

Home remedies for Alcohol Detox #10: Oats***—Avena sativa
· Excellent for weaning off alcohol, drugs, opiates, narcotics. Invigorating without intoxication or overstimulation. Improves clarity, focus.
· Restores proper nerve functioning; eases a racing heart or palpitations.

Home remedies for Alcohol Detox #11: Passionflower*—Passiflora incarnata
· Treats insomnia, delirium tremens or spasms related to withdrawal.
· Useful to induce restful sleep without producing hangover effects.
· Combines well with kava, skullcap, valerian, hops or Jamaican dogwood.

Home remedies for Alcohol Detox #12: Quassia*—Picrasma/Quassia excelsa
· Antidotes effects of alcohol, rejuvenates the spleen. A bitter that stimulates appetite and digestive function; tonifies a weak digestive system.

Home remedies for Alcohol Detox #13: Schisandra**—Schisandra chinensis
· Controls anger and aggression without sedation; combats depression.
· A liver tonic for hepatitis and an adaptogen that assists the body in balancing stress; effective for nervous exhaustion, weakness, insomnia.

Home remedies for Alcohol Detox #14: Wild Lettuce*—Lactuca virosa
· Produces a general sense of well-being, calms excitability, relieves pain.
· Mild sedative and cure for insomnia; safe for both young and old.

Home Remedies for Lupus

Lupus is a chronic autoimmune disease in which the body's immune system attacks its own connective tissue. This causes inflammation and damage to the skin and other organs, and leads to more and more varied infections. Lupus is most frequently a disease of women in their thirties and forties. Genetic factors play a role. In a predisposed person, environmental factors such as a latent viral infection, the use of certain drugs, exposure to ultraviolet light, or bodily injury can provoke the onset of the disease.

Chronic cutaneous lupus erythematosus, or discoid lupus erythematosus (DLE), is a form of the condition in which only the skin is involved. Lupus is generally much less severe than SLE, which can affect not only the skin, but also the kidneys, blood vessels, eyes, lungs, nerves, and joints. Another form of the disease, subacute cutaneous lupus erythematosus (SCLE), is midway in severity between IDLE and SLE. People with SCLE have a psoriasis-like skin rash and may also have joint pains and some blood-count abnormalities. However, they do not have the very serious problems that SLE sufferers can develop.

Typical lesions of Lupus are sharply defined red, scaly patches across the cheeks, nose, and outer ear canals. Other small red, scaly patches may also be seen on sun-exposed sites, such as the arms, legs, scalp, and upper body. Often there are also prominent blood vessels and large follicular openings in these patches. The lesions expand, become white and slightly sunken in the center, and heal with scarring and darkened or lightened pigmentation.

The rash is more common in the summer months, as it tends to flare up in response to sun exposure. Other factors that can make the rash worse include local trauma, menstruation, fatigue, and illness. Persons with Lupus may also suffer from oral and nasal ulcers and permanent hair loss.

Home remedies for Lupus

Home remedies for Lupus #1: Anti-inflammatory herbs that can help to calm the inflammation of lupus include the following:

Home remedies for Lupus #2: Pine bark extract. Take 50 milligrams twice a day

Home remedies for Lupus #3: Grapeseed extract. Take 50 milligrams twice a day

Home remedies for Lupus #4: Turmeric. Take 300 milligrams three times a day.

Home remedies for Lupus #5: Reishi mushroom extract enhances immune function. Take 1 gram (1,000 milligrams) three times a day.

Home remedies for Lupus #6: Avoid the herb echinacea. It stimulates the immune system, and should not be used in an autoimmune disease such as lupus.

Dietary Treatment for Lupus

A low-calorie, low-fat diet, with only limited amounts of beef and dairy products that are high in saturated fat, is recommended.

Have plenty of green raw and steamed vegetables, chicken, and fish. Eating oily fish such as salmon or sardines packed in sardine oil three times a week helps to fight inflammation and heal the skin manifestations of lupus.

Drink eight glasses of pure water every day.

Look for any food sensitivities that may be worsening the disease, and eliminate those foods from the diet. Sensitivities to wheat and chocolate are often involved in causing flare-ups.

Avoid alfalfa, alfalfa seeds, and alfalfa sprouts. These foods contain an immune-stimulating compound, L-canavanine, and also interfere with protein metabolism. Researchers at the Oregon Health Sciences University first found that monkeys eating alfalfa or alfalfa sprouts became sick with a lupus- like infection within six months, the effects of which were partially reversible with the elimination of alfalfa products from their diet. L-canavanine fed directly to monkeys also caused lupus-like symptoms. These same results have been seen in individuals who eat large quantities of alfalfa products.

Avoid plants in the nightshade family, including tomatoes, eggplant, and peppers. These can also make the symptoms of lupus worse.

Eliminate from your diet animal fats and oils high in omega-6 oils, such as corn, safflower, and sunflower oils. These promote inflammation.

Psoriasis is among the most common and most difficult to control of all skin diseases, affecting about 2 percent of the population. It affects men and women equally, and usually appears between the ages of fifteen and thirty. It generally follows a chronic course of acute flare-ups alternating with periods of remission.

The word psoriasis is derived from the Greek psora, which means "to itch." Salmon-red bumps with a silvery scale appear on the skin, get bigger, and grow together to form large plaques. Lesions of psoriasis vary in size from fractions of an inch in diameter to large plaques covering most of the body and requiring hospitalization. Places on the body most commonly affected by psoriasis include the elbows, knees, scalp, and sacral areas. The nails are involved in about one-half of cases, with pitting, breaking, thickening under the nail, or thickening of the nail itself. In addition, between 10 and 30 percent of people with psoriasis also suffer from psoriatic arthritis, which can be quite painful.

Because of the chronic, difficult nature of psoriasis, professional help is needed in all but the least severe cases.

There appear to be many reasons why some people develop psoriasis and others do not. It has a tendency to be inherited—about one-third of those who have it have another family member with psoriasis. Several studies have documented the relationship between specific stresses and the start and flare-ups of psoriasis. Almost half of all people with psoriasis report that a specific stressful event occurred within one month before the first episode of psoriasis.

Home remedies for Psoriasis

Home remedies for Psoriasis #1: Herbal liver tonics, together with tissue and blood cleansers, or alteratives, form the most important initial part of herbal treatment for psoriasis. Slightly less important are nerve tonics, or nervines, which soothe the nerves and lessen the itching of psoriasis.

Home remedies for Psoriasis #2: Applying aloe vera gel to the lesions can help. Dr. Andrew Weil reported that 83 percent of psoriasis patients who applied aloe-vera cream three times a day for up to four weeks noted an improvement. Dr. Weil recommends using pure aloe vera gel instead of an aloe vera cream that contains other ingredients.

Home remedies for Psoriasis #3: Apple-cider vinegar diluted in water can be used to temporarily help relieve itching and scaling. Apple cider vinegar or white vinegar can also be diluted in three to four times as much lukewarm water and poured over the head, rubbed in, left for one minute, and then rinsed out. Or you can add 1/2 cup of cider vinegar to a tubful of bath water to help restore acidity to the skin.

Home remedies for Psoriasis #4: Banana peel is a key ingredient in Exorex. This is a lotion concocted from coal tar and a specific essential fatty acid from banana peel that is associated with the immune system. Reportedly, the idea was derived from Zulu folklore, in which banana peels have been used for a variety of skin ailments for years.

Home remedies for Psoriasis #5: Burdock root can help improve flare-ups of psoriasis. Take 20 to 40 drops of tincture three times a day.

Home remedies for Psoriasis #6: Chamomile is widely used in Europe for treating psoriasis. It contains anti-inflammatory flavonoid compounds. If you have ragweed allergies, however, do not use chamomile, as it is a member of the ragweed family.

Home remedies for Psoriasis #7: Castor oil is particularly helpful when left overnight on thick, small, well-circumscribed lesions. If cold-pressed castor oil is mixed with baking soda, it has been found to greatly improve thick, scaly heel skin, as long as the skin isn't cracked.

Home remedies for Psoriasis #8: Cayenne pepper has anti-inflammatory properties and helps with healing. Two clinical trials reviewed in the November 1998 issue of Archives of Dermatology reported that 0.025 percent capsaicin cream, made from hot peppers, works to reduce the redness and scaling in psoriasis. Capsaicin cream is available over the counter as Capzasin-P or Zostrix. It should be used over a six-week period. Care should be taken not to apply it to broken skin.

Home remedies for Psoriasis #9: Common figwort helps to clear psoriatic plaques. The recommended dose is 2 milliliters of tincture, taken twice a day.

Home remedies for Psoriasis #10: Dandelion tincture is useful for stimulating bile flow and clearing toxins out of the system. It is frequently combined with yellow dock (see below) for this purpose. The recommended dose is 30 to 60 drops twice a day.

Home remedies for Psoriasis #11: Echinacea tincture is occasionally used for psoriasis. It boosts the immune system, and so may decrease the incidence of colds, which can lead to flare-ups in some individuals. The recommended dose is 20 to 30 drops three times a day for up to ten days. Stop for two weeks, then repeat.

Home remedies for Psoriasis #12: Emu oil contains essential fatty acids and may be helpful for psoriasis. Apply it to the lesions as directed by the manufacturer.

Home remedies for Psoriasis #13: Flaxseed oil is chemically similar to fish oil and helps treat psoriasis. Adding flaxseed oil to salad dressing is a good way to get this helpful supplement into your diet. Take 1½2 tablespoons of flaxseed oil daily.

Home remedies for Psoriasis #14: Fumitory contains fumaric acid, which has been found to be very helpful for psoriasis. Make a strong tea from fumitory and apply it to the affected areas with a cotton ball twice a day.

Home remedies for Psoriasis #15: Garlic is detoxifying and includes a number of sulfur-containing compounds. Sulfur deficiency may contribute to psoriasis. Take three to six garlic capsules daily.

Home remedies for Psoriasis #16: Goldenseal tincture helps to clear the body of toxins that lead to flareups. Take 20 to 30 drops twice a day for up to ten days at a time.

Home remedies for Psoriasis #17: Gotu kola extract reduces inflammation and speeds skin healing. In India, it has been used for psoriasis for hundreds of years. Take 200 milligrams three times a day for one month.

Home remedies for Psoriasis #18: Liquid licorice extract, applied directly to the affected areas with a cotton ball, is felt by some naturopaths to work as well as corticosteroid creams.

Home remedies for Psoriasis #19: Flaxseed oil, applied to affected areas twice a day, is said to help heal psoriasis. Avocado, garlic, and walnut oils, applied topically twice a day to the psoriatic patches, are equally helpful for moisturizing and healing.

Home remedies for Psoriasis #20: Milk thistle cleanses and protects the liver, increases bile flow, and helps in blood purification. It also helps to correct the abnormal cell replication present in psoriasis. Take 300 milligrams of milk-thistle extract three times a day.

Home remedies for Psoriasis #21: Neem-seed oil, an Ayurvedic herbal remedy, is highly recommended by some psoriasis sufferers. It was introduced to the United States in 1994 from India and Pakistan. Neem lotions are usually found in East Indian markets

Home Remedies for Itching

Itching is a superficial sensation in the skin, probably originating at the border between the epidermis and the dermis. Histamine, a body chemical released in response to contact with an irritant of some kind, is thought to be one of the most common triggers for itching, although there are other chemical mediators in the skin and blood.

There are many causes of itching. Common causes of acute itching include allergies to plants, pollens, cats, dogs, feathers, perfumes, cosmetics, cleaning solutions, other chemicals, and smoke. Short-lived skin problems such as very dry skin, fungal infection, lice, scabies, and sunburn are also frequent reasons for itching. Pregnancy can sometimes produce itching and related skin problems.

Home remedies for Itching

Home remedies for Itching #1: A paste made from aloe vera gel and green clay soothes the skin.

Home remedies for Itching #2: Chamomile cream, calendula lotion, or comfrey ointment can be applied directly to the itchy areas as often as needed. They have anti-inflammatory properties that help to relieve your discomfort.

Home remedies for Itching #3: Jewelweed, otherwise known as impatiens, can be boiled in a gallon of water, strained and cooled. The liquid stops itching extremely well. In fact, in clinical trials, it worked just as well as prescription cortisone creams. Jewelweed is a perennial wildflower that should be available at herb shops and through herbalists. It is not the same plant as the flowering annual called impatiens that is commonly sold in nurseries and garden centers.

Home remedies for Itching #4: An herbal tea made from two parts each of agrimony and chamomile and one part each of stinging nettle and heart's-ease can be taken three times a day as an aid to soothing the itching. In addition to drinking the tea, dip a clean cloth into it and apply it as a compress to the affected areas for five minutes every half hour, as needed. Other plants containing naturally antihistaminic compounds from which you can make a combination tea include basil, fennel, ginkgo, oregano, tarragon, tea, thyme, and yarrow. These teas should be used to compress the affected areas of itchy skin, as well as drunk three times a day

Home remedies for Itching #5: Diluted chamomile, lavender, and rosemary essential oils are soothing and relaxing, and help ease itching. You can add up to 10 drops of any of these oils (or a combination) to a tubful of water to make an aromatherapy bath, or you can dilute them in a carrier oil such as jojoba oil and apply it to the hives with a compress.

Home remedies for Itching #6: Rhus toxicodendron 30x or 15c is recommended for itching, especially if it is accompanied by joint pain or fever, or if discomfort is worse with the cold or scratching. Take one dose four times a day, up to a total of eight doses.

Home Remedies For Rash

An inflammation of the skin, is used to describe many different types of rashes. The skin may itch, flake, scale, thicken, ooze, crust, and/or redden, depending on the type of dermatitis. Rashes can develop anywhere on the body. Certain locations are typical for different forms of rashes.

Atopic dermatitis, or eczema, the "itch that rashes" is a chronic, common problem that affects many people and for which there are many possible therapies. It is discussed in its own section (see Eczema). Contact dermatitis is probably the most common type of dermatitis. It is caused by irritation or allergy to something the skin comes in contact with. Types of rashes include irritant contact dermatitis, allergic contact dermatitis, and photoallergic contact dermatitis. A common type of allergic contact dermatitis is the rash of poison ivy, oak, and sumac. These also are described in their own section (see Poison Ivy, Oak, and Sumac).

Seborrhea (seborrheic dermatitis) is another distinct type of rash, and is discussed in its own section as well.

Home remedies for Rash

Home remedies for Rash #1: · Naturopaths believe that when waste products build up and exceed the capacity of the liver and kidneys to get rid of them, the skin has to eliminate the wastes. This can result in dermatitis. The following herbs cause sweating, which naturopaths feel is a good way to excrete the toxins that are trying to get out of your body:

Home remedies for Rash #2: Burdock root. Take 500 milligrams three times a day, with meals.

Home remedies for Rash #3: Sarsaprilla root. Take it as directed by the manufacturer.

Home remedies for Rash #4: Yarrow. Take it as directed by the manufacturer.

Naturopaths recommend one or more of the follow blood cleansers for rash:

Home remedies for Rash #5: Chaparral root. Take it as directed by the manufacturer.

Home remedies for Rash #6: Dandelion root. Take it as directed by the manufacturer.

Home remedies for Rash #7: Echinacea. Take it as directed by the manufacturer.

Home remedies for Rash #8: Goldenseal. Take 500 milligrams three times a day, with meals.

Home remedies for Rash #9: Pau d'arco. Take 500 milligrams three times a day, with meals.

Home remedies for Rash #10: Poke root. Make a tea by steeping 1 tablespoon of the herb in a cup of water. Drink this twice a day.

Home remedies for Rash #11: Red clover. Take 500 milligrams three times a day.

Home remedies for Rash #12: Yellow dock root. Take it as directed by the manufacturer.

Home remedies for Rash #13: The appropriate specific herbal therapy depends on the cause, location, and type of rash. However, the following therapies will all help relieve itching, no matter what sort of dermatitis you have:

Home remedies for Rash #14: Aloe vera gel and green clay soothe the skin.

Home remedies for Rash #15: Chamomile cream, calendula lotion, or comfrey ointment should be applied directly to the itchy areas as often as needed, as their anti-inflammatory properties will help relieve your discomfort.

Home remedies for Rash #16: Chickweed infusion can be used to bathe the area to stop itching.

Home remedies for Rash #17: Cucumber puree, made from peeled, blended fresh cucumbers, can be applied directly to the affected area for three minutes to relieve your itching and pain.

Home remedies for Rash #18: Jewelweed, also known as impatiens, can be boiled in a gallon of water, strained, and cooled. The liquid stops itching extremely well. In fact, in clinical trials, it has worked just as well as prescription cortisone creams. Note that while it is sometimes called impatiens, jewelweed is not the same plant that is sold as a flowering annual in home and garden centers.

Home remedies for Rash #19: An herbal tea made from two parts each of agrimony and chamomile and one part each of stinging nettle and heart's-ease can be taken three times a day as an aid to soothing the itching. In addition to drinking the tea, dip a clean cloth into it and apply it as a compress to the affected areas for five minutes every half hour, as needed. Other plants containing natural antihistaminic compounds from which you can make a combination tea include basil, fennel, ginkgo, oregano, tarragon, tea, thyme, and yarrow. These teas should be used in compresses applied to the itchy areas, as well as drunk three times a day.

Ringworm or tinea, is a fungal infection growing on the outer layers of the skin, scalp, and/or nails. Athlete's foot and "jock itch" are actually localized forms of ringworm. Other favored sites of fungal infection are the palms and soles, nails, scalp, beard, and trunk.

Fungal infections are rapidly spread from one person to another or even from the family pet to the family. They recur often, and when they do, they have to be treated again.

Fungal infections on the body usually start as itchy, slightly scaly, round red spots on the skin. As the lesions grow, they heal from the inside of the round circle out, giving the rash its characteristic ringlike appearance. The infection often spreads from one area of the body to another. If your groin is involved, there is usually a diffuse red, scaling rash that is very itchy. If you have tinea of your palms or feet, they often scale and are red and may blister, but do not usually form separate small spots. Nail infections appear as areas of yellowish or whitish discoloration and crumbling. Scalp infection with ringworm produces red, itchy scaling and, later, hair loss and breakage.

Doctors confirm a diagnosis of tinea by looking at some of the skin scales under a microscope to see if fungal bodies are present. Generally, treatment is very effective and relatively quick, and there are many good options. Therapy takes longer if the fungi have been invading the scalp, fingernails, or toenails for some time.

Home remedies for Ringworm

Home remedies for Ringworm #1: Calendula cream, ointment, or tincture diluted in warm water has anti- fungal, astringent, and healing properties, and can be used two to three times a day as an aid in fighting fungal infections of the body

Home remedies for Ringworm #2: Chamomile tea, taken three times a day, should help clear ringworm. It can also be applied directly to the affected areas with a cotton ball three times a day

Home remedies for Ringworm #3: Garlic is one of the best herbal antifungals. Its antifungal properties have been documented by clinical studies showing that the blood of people taking garlic has significant antifungal activity. Take 6 teaspoons of garlic extract daily. In addition, you can put raw garlic in a blender and apply the resulting paste to areas of ringworm with a clean cotton ball three times a day

Home remedies for Ringworm #4: Ginger tea, made by simmering 2 ounces of fresh ginger root simmered in 8 ounces of water for twenty minutes, contains more than twenty anti- fungal compounds. Drink the tea three times a day and also apply a compress consisting of cotton soaked with the ginger tea to the affected areas for five minutes three times a day.

Home remedies for Ringworm #5: Goldenseal is another good antifungal agent. Add 5 drops of the tincture to juice and drink it three times a day. Or simmer 6 teaspoons of the dried herb for twenty minutes to make a tea, strain out the herbal matter, and apply the tea to your areas of tinea three times a day with a fresh cotton ball. You can also dust your feet, socks, and shoes with goldenseal powder twice a day.

Home remedies for Ringworm #6: Take a cup of lemongrass tea three times a day. While you drink the tea, apply the used tea bags to the affected areas. This should help ringworm to clear faster.

Home remedies for Ringworm #7: Licorice contains at least twenty-five fungicidal substances. Add 6 teaspoons of powdered licorice root to a cup of boiling water and simmer for twenty minutes. Strain out the herbal matter, and apply the tea to the areas of ringworm three times a day using a fresh cotton ball.

Home remedies for Ringworm #8: Myrrh is a good antifungal. Make a paste by mixing equal parts of myrrh and goldenseal powder with a little water, and apply it to the areas of rash three times a day.

Home remedies for Ringworm #9: Olive-leaf extract has antifungal properties and helps to fortify the immune system. Take 250 milligrams three times a day.

Anti Aging Remedies

Life span is ultimately determined by the fact that cells can only replicate a certain number of times—a genetically predetermined cut-off point that prevents physical immortality. Understanding this, most researchers still believe that humans should live 120 years or more. Why then is the average life span hovering around age 70? We deteriorate mainly due to damage from free radicals, produced as a byproduct of normal metabolism, or created by various toxins, pollutants, allergens, heavy metals, etc. Additionally, 75% of Americans are not getting enough free radical fighting antioxidants, such as vitamin E, selenium or even vitamin C. These are quickly used up under stress, while hormonal, immune and neurological imbalances further accelerate aging.

A number of herbs are highly prized and renowned for their anti-aging and longevity-promoting effects. Science has extensively verified that these complex plant medicines have the definite ability to prolong the duration and quality of life. Many of these anti-aging herbs are adaptogens and tonics, normalizing metabolic, hormonal and neurological systems and stimulating cellular regeneration. Others have more focused effects on the brain, heart or immunity. They are safe for long-term use and disease prevention. See also Immune Weakness - Memory - Stress.

Anti Aging Remedies

Anti Aging Remedies #1: Ashwaganda***—Withania somnifera
· Tonic that slows aging, rejuvenates tissues throughout the body.
· Clears the mind, strengthens the nerves, promotes restful sleep.
· Improves memory, cholesterol, sexual ability; lessens hair graying.

Anti Aging Remedies #2: Fo-Ti***—Polygonum multiflorum
· Chinese tonic herb that promotes longevity, strengthens the blood, improves vitality, sexual vigor and fertility and can reduce hair graying.
· Lowers cholesterol, improves arteriosclerosis, regulates blood sugar.

Anti Aging Remedies #3: Garlic**—Allium sativa
· Protects nervous system, improves brain function, memory, learning.
· Prevents/treats arteriosclerosis, reduces clotting, lowers cholesterol.
· Increases life span in animal tests; inhibits viruses, bacteria, parasites.

Anti Aging Remedies #4: Ginseng* * *—Panax ginseng
· Rejuvenating, stimulating adaptogen, yet helps calm nerves, increases vitality; reduces exhaustion; increases stamina, speeds wound healing.
· Enhances immune system; balances metabolism and stress response.

Anti Aging Remedies #5: Gotu Kola***—Centella asiatica
· Rejuvenating, longevity herb in the Ayurvedic and Chinese traditions.
· Increases intelligence, memory, creativity, learning ability, reduces mental fatigue. Strengthens nervous system, adrenals and immune system.
· Improves wound healing, reduces scar tissue, increases circulation.

Anti Aging Remedies #6: Green Tea**—Camellia sinensis
· High in vitamins, minerals, antioxidants and flavonoids and especially polyphenols; decreases cellular and tissue damage incurred with aging.
· Protective against cancer, heart diseases and is an immune stimulant.

Anti Aging Remedies #7: Hawthorn**—Crataegus oxycantha
· Heart and circulation tonic; normalizes blood pressure, heart rhythm.
· Slows aging process, protects connective tissue and blood vessel walls.
· Reduces atherosclerosis, helps adaptation to physical and mental stress, protects against radiation, improves digestion and assimilation.

Anti Aging Remedies #8: Licorice**—Glycyrrhiza glabra
· Traditional Chinese longevity herb; stimulates adrenal glands, balances and conserves cortisol and energy during stress. Anti-inflammatory.
· Has potent antioxidants that protect the digestive tract, liver and other tissues from the damaging effects of aging. Inhibits atrophy of thymus.

Anti Aging Remedies #9: Maca**—Lepidium meyenii
· Ancient Peruvian herb that increases vitality, strength and stamina.
· Invigorates libido and is a sexual restorative in both men and women.
· Alleviates signs of decreasing hormones in middle age and menopause.

Anti Aging Remedies #10: Reishi***—Ganoderma lucida
· A traditional "elixir of immortality" in Traditional Chinese Medicine.
· Treats a wide range of conditions, including heart disease and cancer.
· Normalizes blood pressure, cholesterol, platelet stickiness. Enhances immune and liver health, helps indigestion, eases tension, improves sleep.

Anti Aging Remedies #11: Rhodiola**—Golden Root/Rhodiola rosea
· Increases immunity, prolongs life span, increases exercise capacity.
· Clears toxins, strengthens nervous and digestive system. Reduces fatigue.

Anti Aging Remedies #12: Siberian Ginseng**—Eleuthrococcus senticosus
· Called the "king of adaptogens," has a wide range of vitalizing effects.
· Increases hearing, improves eyesight, supports immunity and stress adaptation. Increases mental and physical work capacity.

Anti Aging Remedies #13: Suma**—Pfaffia paniculata
· An adaptogen that is antiviral, antibacterial and immune stimulating.
· Increases muscle mass, protein production, overall physical endurance.
· Balances hormones, reduces blood sugar, cholesterol, triglycerides.
· Reduces fatigue, promotes liver and kidney regeneration, skin healing.

Home Remedies For backache

backache affects at least 80% of people at some time, and most often concentrates in the low back. This results in an estimated 40 million days of lost work, at a cost of $70 billion. Poor postural habits are a major contributing cause, while other factors include repeated strains or microtrauma, muscle tension, nutritional deficiencies and reflex irritation from related internal organs. When repeated episodes of injury are added to this mix, the discs become subject to thinning, deterioration or rupture. These events can also gradually lead to arthritic changes.

With nerves close by, swelling or compression in the spine often results in neuritis, lumbar neuralgia or sciatica.

Herbal medicines are used similarly to medical drugs in this type of condition, though with far more safety. Both the anti-inflammatory and pain-relieving qualities of plants can be used effectively and taken for prolonged periods of time. Other benefits are relief of muscle spasm and repair of connective tissue and cartilage tissue. Bioflavonoids and other healing factors contained in herbs, along with well-known nutritional substances like glucosamine sulphate, can complete deeper repair and strengthening of tissues. The herbs listed under Arthritis can provide further help for chronic joint dysfunction. If nerves become inflamed or compressed, additional sedative and nerve-repairing herbs may be needed. See also Arthritis

Use These Home Remedies for backache

Home Remedies for backache #1: Barberry* *—Berberis vulgaris
· For low backache, often related to kidney weakness or congestion.
· For sciatica and neuralgia with radiating pain and weakened muscles
· Use in rheumatic disorders, sciatica, bursitis, neuralgia and gout.

Home Remedies for backache #2: Black Cohosh**—Cimicifuga racemosa
· Anti-inflammatory effects, relaxing muscle spasms in low back and neck.
· Suitable for wry neck (torticollis), sciatica, neuralgia and intercostal (rib) neuralgia. Treats muscle pain associated with fibromyalgia, arthritis.

Home Remedies for backache #3: Black Haw***—Viburnum prunifolia
· With aspirin-like ingredients, relieves spasms and neuralgia of back and neck, sciatica, leg cramps, tension headache, wry neck, digestive spasm.
· A nervous system tonic and sedative, helps backache during menses.

Home Remedies for backache #4: Boswellia***—Boswellia serrata
· Strong anti-inflammatory effects, reduces stiffness and pain.
· Works for acute problems, but needs 2-4 weeks for maximal effects.
· Improves circulation around inflamed joints, ligaments, tendons.

Home Remedies for backache #5: Bromelain**—Pineapple/Ananas comosus
· Enzyme found in pineapple stem, helps resolve late stages of inflammation, speeding healing and reducing the potential for scar tissue.

Home Remedies for backache #6: Corydalis*—Corydalis soldida
· Chinese herb that relieves pain of all kinds, especially from injury.
· Sedative, analgesic, relives spasm and abdominal pain, dysmenorrhea.
· Often used in combination with other complementary herbs.

Home Remedies for backache #7: Devil's Claw**—Harpagophytum procumbens
· Anti-inflammatory and pain-relieving herb, with rapid results.
· Useful for low backache, arthritis and chronic rheumatic disorders, neuralgia and headaches. The whole herb preparation works best.

Home Remedies for backache #8: Dong Quai**—Angelica sinensis
· Reported to possess 1.5 times the analgesic activity of aspirin.
· Relieves backache, cramping, muscular spasms and inflammation.
· Also for menstrual cycle regulation, anemia; a liver and heart tonic.

Home Remedies for backache #9: Horse Chestnut*—Aesculus hippocastanum
· Low back, sacrum, and sacroiliac pain. Stiff, weak back that "gives out."
· Helps with arthritic and rheumatic backache with heaviness, swelling.

Home Remedies for backache #10: Jamaican Dogwood***—Piscidia erythrina
· Strong sedative, pain-relieving and antispasmodic effects.
· Especially valuable for muscular back spasms and pain, but also used in asthma, menstrual pain, insomnia, toothache or nervous conditions.

Home Remedies for backache #11: Kava Kava**—Piper methysticum
· Relaxes muscles, reduces internal and external spasms and cramps.
· Pain reliever, plus enhances pain-reducing effects of aspirin and drugs.
· No hangover, tolerance, build-up or addiction, typical of medical drugs.

Home Remedies for backache #12: Meadowsweet*—Filipendula ulmaria
· Herbal forerunner of aspirin provides anti-inflammatory pain relief.
· No gastric irritation like medical NSAIDs; neutralizes stomach acids and general internal acidity.

Home Remedies for backache #13: Valerian**—Valeriana officinalis
· Relaxing and sedative effects, reduces transmission of pain signals.
· Muscle relaxant, relieves muscle spasms and contractures due to stress and tension; eases menstrual pain, colic, asthma, irritable bowel spasm.

Home Remedies for backache #14: Wild Yam**—Dioscorea villosa
· Indicated for backache characterized by sharp, knife-like sensations.
· A relaxant used for pain originating in the digestive system, gall bladder, nervous system, uterus. Supplies precursors for adrenal cortisol.

Arteriosclerosis or hardening of the arteries is the leading cause of disease and death in America, causing heart disease, stroke, kidney disease and problems with circulation in the limbs.

Arteriosclerosis occurs due to oxidative damage to the lining of the arteries, infiltration with fat-filled cells and formation of plaques and clots.

Risk factors include smoking, blood sugar disorders, obesity, an excess of "bad" cholesterol or LDL and high homocysteine levels, as well as a diet high in refined carbohydrates and trans fatty acids (i.e. processed oils). Damage to the arterial wall may also be due to chronic viral or bacterial infection.

Supplementation with folic acid, B12 and B6, CoO10, selenium, omega 3 oils and antioxidants would cut the risk of Arteriosclerosis and heart disease to a fraction of its current rate.

Herbal treatment for hardening of the arteries relies upon the strong antioxidant power of many plants, preventing the arterial damage that acts as a site for the development of plaque. They also prevent oxidation of LDL cholesterol, which leads to arterial deposits. Some herbs can remove existing arteriosclerosis, returning elasticity to arteries. Such plants have multiple benefits, such as toning the heart, reducing cholesterol and preventing blood cell clumping and clot formation. The central herb for the heart is hawthorn, while a combination or rotating schedule of several other healing plants will maximize their long-term benefit.

Home remedies for Arteriosclerosis

Home remedies for Arteriosclerosis #1: Arjuna**—Terminalia arjuna
· Main Ayurvedic heart tonic, normalizes the heart's rhythm, improves blood flow in coronary arteries. Reduces cholesterol; antibacterial.
· Improves symptoms of congestive heart failure and reduces angina pain.

Home remedies for Arteriosclerosis #2: Bromelain**—Pineapple/Ananas comosus
· A proteolytic enzyme derived from the stem of the pineapple plant.
· Reduces blood platelet "stickiness" and subsequent clot formation.
· Decreases the inflammatory response to artery injury or irritation.

Home remedies for Arteriosclerosis #3: Cayenne**—Capsicum frutescens
· Stimulates blood flow, lowers cholesterol; may affect arteriosclerosis.
· Reduces risk of blood clotting, increases heart output.
· Increases capillary resistance, strengthens blood vessels in the limbs.
· Improves peripheral circulation and warms the hands and feet.

Home remedies for Arteriosclerosis #4: Curcamin***—Turmeric/Curcuma longa
· Antioxidant power eight times more potent than Vitamin E; prevents damage to blood vessel walls to prevent onset of arteriosclerosis.

· Improves blood flow in arteries, while strengthening blood vessels.
· Significantly reduces cholesterol, serum lipids, blood clot formation.

Home remedies for Arteriosclerosis #5: Garlic ***—Allium sativa
· In one two-year study, reduced the size of arterial plaque by 20%.
· Blocks the formation of new plaque.
· Lowers cholesterol and triglycerides (by 10-20%), lowers LDL and raises HDL cholesterol; prevents oxidation and thus damage to arteries.
· A natural anti-coagulant; helps dissolve potential clots (fibrinolysis).

Home remedies for Arteriosclerosis #6: Ginger* *—Zingiber officinale
· Thins the blood, decreases platelet aggregation and lowers cholesterol.
· Decreases blood pressure and reduces hardening of the arteries.
· Antioxidant, contains potent proteolytic enzymes; prevents clots.

Home remedies for Arteriosclerosis #7: Ginkgo***—Ginkgo biloba
· Increases microcirculation to all parts of the body, heart, limbs, brain.
· Blood-thinning activity, inhibits clot formation and inflammation.
· Antioxidant; strengthens, tones arteries, improving their elasticity.

Home remedies for Arteriosclerosis #8: Grape Seed Extract***—Vitis vinifera
· Antioxidant power 20 times that of vitamin C, 50 times vitamin E.
· Prevents arteriosclerosis and improves circulation in arteries, veins.
· Lowers cholesterol and actually shrinks existing deposits in arteries.
· Reduces blood cell agglutination, preventing clots, heart attack, stroke.
· Proanthocyanidins (OPCs) strengthen vessel walls, capillaries.

Home remedies for Arteriosclerosis #9: Guggul***—Commiphora gulgul
· Prevents arteriosclerosis, while reducing existing plaque in arteries.
· Lowers cholesterol and triglycerides as well as medical drugs. Lowers total cholesterol up to 30% in 3 months, raising HDL and lowering LDL.

Home remedies for Arteriosclerosis #10: Hawthorn***—Crataegus oxycantha
Traditionally used over a long term to remove arteriosclerotic deposits.
· Essential cardiotonic that strengthens the heart muscle (myocardium).
· Prevents cardiovascular disease by dilating the coronary vessels.
· Improves blood and oxygen to the heart, coronary arteries and tissues.
· Strengthens contraction of the heart muscles, regulates blood pressure.

Home remedies for Arteriosclerosis #11: Shlitake**—Lentinus edodes
· Protective antioxidant, inhibits the formation of arteriosclerotic plaque.
· Helps prevent cardiovascular disease, stroke and diabetes.
· Lowers cholesterol up to 15%, prevents clots, regulates blood sugar.

The term UTI includes bladder irritation, as well as infection caused by various microorganisms.

Bladder infection conditions occur more often in women, due to anatomical differences. In middle-aged men, however, a swollen prostate is the typical cause for urinary retention and infection. Underlying causes include nutritional deficiencies and immune susceptibility, as well as the more obvious irritations from intercourse, tight clothing, spices, coffee, tea, medicines, alcohol or high sugar in the urine. Food allergies may be a significant factor, especially in children.

Herbs for the urinary tract infection generally have diuretic effects, to flush out infection and inflammation by-products. Many are also antimicrobial, either destroying microorganisms or stimulating the body to do so. Along with quelling inflammation, other plants help heal irritated mucus membrane linings of the bladder, urethra and ureter, and the kidney tubules.

In most cases, simple bladder infection can be easily and effectively dealt with using the herbs below. In cases where antibiotic resistant bacteria are involved, or where no bacteria are detected, as in interstitial cystitis, herbs become even more important and uniquely effective.

Home remedies for bladder Infection

Home remedies for bladder Infection #1: Buchu**—Agathosma or Barosma betulina
· A diuretic and urinary antiseptic for cystitis, urethritis, prostatitis.
· Tones the urinary tract and helps prevent stones; treats bedwetting.
· Helpful for prostate enlargement and resulting bladder infections.

Home remedies for bladder Infection #2: Corn Silk**—Zea mays
· A soothing diuretic for irritation of the bladder, urethra and prostate.
· Relieves urinary tract inflammation and bedwetting in children.
· Effective for difficult and scant urination, cystitis and kidney stones.

Home remedies for bladder Infection #2: Couchgrass*—Agropyron repens
· A soothing urinary demulcent, useful for infection or inflammation of the prostate, urethra or bladder. Useful in kidney stone and gravel.

Home remedies for bladder Infection #3: Cranberry***—Vacciniurn macrocarpon
· Reduces bacteria and prevents them from adhering to the bladder walls.
· Can be taken as a preventive in people with recurring infections.
· Safe and effective during pregnancy, for children and the elderly.
· Mildly acidifies the urine, eliminating alkaline bacteria, (i.e. E. coli).
· Reduces effectiveness of uva ursi; should not be used together.

Home remedies for bladder Infection #4: Goldenrod**—Solidago virgaurea
Diuretic, anti-inflammatory and antiseptic effects for cystitis, urethritis.

Pain-relieving and antifungal, tones the bladder, soothes irritation. Safe and mild action; does not deplete body's electrolytes/potassium.

Home remedies for bladder Infection #5: Goldenseal***—Hydrastis canadensis
Anti-inflammatory and antimicrobial; destroys many types of bacteria.
· Especially effective for chronic cystitis or stubborn urinary mucus.
· Healing effect on bladder linings, stops bleeding, heals ulcerations.

Home remedies for bladder Infection #6: Gravel Root—Joe Pye Weed/Eupatorium purpureum
For bedwetting in kids with bad dreams, hold their urine in too long. ® For irritable bladder with frequent desire, always feels full, uneasy.
For incontinence in women, old age, children, enlarged prostate.

Home remedies for bladder Infection #7: Horsetail**—Equisetum arvense
Acute urinary tract infection; safe during pregnancy or weakened states. For bed-wetting or enuresis in children or weak bladder in the elderly.
Diuretic effects, but does not deplete the body of salts or electrolytes.

Home remedies for bladder Infection #8: Juniper Berry*—Juniperus communis
A powerful diuretic, antispasmodic and strong antibiotic for cystitis.
▪ Must not be used for prolonged periods or in kidney infections.

Home remedies for bladder Infection #9: Marshmallow***—Althea officinalis
A soothing demulcent to the lining of the urinary tract.
Use for acute inflammation, typical of bladder infections.
Decreases inflammation in the respiratory, digestive or urinary tract.

Home remedies for bladder Infection #10: Parsley Root*—Petroselinum crispum
Diuretic effects for cystitis, kidney stones. Soothes burning, itching, crawling in the urethra. Avoid in kidney disease or pregnancy.
Helps symptoms of pain, frequent desire, urging, mucus discharges.

Home remedies for bladder Infection #11: Sarsaparilla***—Smilax officinalis
For cystitis, kidney infections, bladder stones, kidney colic, bedwetting. " A blood purifier that is antiseptic, anti-inflammatory; controls itching.
Diuretic. Rheumatic or skin problems (psoriasis) with urinary irritation.

Home remedies for bladder Infection #12: Uva ursi***—Arctostaphylos uva ursi
Urinary disinfectant and antiseptic, effective for many types of bacteria. " Diuretic and astringent for chronic and acute urinary problems. " Avoid acidic foods—and cranberry—which decrease its effectiveness.

Home remedies for bladder Infection #13: Yarrow**—Achillea millefolium
Increases urination, has antimicrobial effects, stops bleeding. Anti-inflammatory properties, while soothing bladder spasms. Tones the urinary tract and acts as a mild pain reliever in infections.

Home Remedies Bad Breath

Bad breath is an embarrassing problem. A person with bad breath may be offensive without realizing it, as all the advertisements for breath mints, mouthwashes, and toothpastes are so quick to point out. In some cases, an unusual breath odor may be a sign of illness, such as a herpes infection of the mouth, diabetes, postnasal drip, tonsillitis, sinusitis, dental infection, strep throat, liver or kidney failure, or a lung abscess. Most of the time, however, bad breath—medically termed halitosis—is not the result of any major health problem. It is usually related to poor oral hygiene or poor digestion, sometimes both.

If a friend or family member (or you yourself) notice a bad smell on your breath, especially if the breath has a persistent or unusual odor, consult your physician. He or she will be able to determine whether or not your bad breath is related to an underlying infection or other illness. One particularly helpful—though, unfortunately, not often recommended—diagnostic test is a comprehensive stool analysis, which can be used to determine problems with digestion and assimilation, the presence of parasites, or the overgrowth of abnormal bacteria in the digestive tract.

Home Remedies for Bad Breath

Bad Breath Home Remedies #1: Take an acidophilus and bifidobacteria supplement daily to establish and maintain favorable intestinal flora and healthy digestion. If you are allergic to milk, select a dairy-free product.

Bad Breath Home Remedies #2: Chlorophyll tablets help freshen the breath because they have a cleansing effect in the intestines. Take a chlorophyll supplement, as directed on the product label, after each meal and again at bedtime.

Bad Breath Home Remedies #3: If you suspect bad breath related to poor digestion, try supplementing your diet with digestive enzymes. There are a number of over-the-counter products available that use natural enzymes—bromelain (from pineapple) or papain (from papaya)—which may be helpful. Follow the dosage directions on the product label.

Bad Breath Home Remedies #4: Sometimes bad breath is a result of poor stomach function. To strengthen the gastrointestinal tract, you may want to try taking duodenal extract with vitamin A as directed on the product label.

Bad Breath Home Remedies #5: Choose an herbal-based toothpaste or tooth powder formulated without sugar. If this type of product is not available in your local drugstore, check a health-food store. Merfluan is a baking-soda-based tooth powder that is very popular in Europe. It comes in several different flavors.

Bad Breath Home Remedies #6: The Chinese patent medicine Fare You is a cabbage extract that helps to heal and strengthen the stomach lining. If bad breath originates from compromised stomach function, consider trying Fare You. Follow the dosage directions on the product label.

Bad Breath Home Remedies #7: Chew on a small sprig of parsley to freshen your breath. Parsley is rich in the natural deodorizer chlorophyll, and also sweetens the digestive tract.

Bad Breath Home Remedies #8: If bad breath is an occasional problem related to poor digestion, typically accompanied by upset stomach, diarrhea, constipation, or a lot of burping, sipping a cup of peppermint tea after meals should help to ease digestion. Or try taking a cup of ginger tea twice a day, with meals, to enhance digestion.

Home Remedies Indigestion

NUTRITIONAL SUPPLEMENTS FOR INDIGESTION

Indigestion Home Remedies #1: Many people with acid reflux find their symptoms improve if they take supplements containing betaine hydrochloride (HC1). Apparently, if the level of acid in the stomach is too low, the sphincter muscle separating the stomach and the esophagus can loosen, allowing what acid there is to escape up into the esophagus. Betaine HC1 increases the acidity of the stomach and helps prevent this problem. It is available in a variety of formulas, both on its own and with additional digestive enzymes. Follow the dosage directions on the product label and take it immediately after meals.

Indigestion Home Remedies #2: If your main complaint occurs within thirty minutes of eating, take a full-spectrum digestive-enzyme supplement providing 5,000 international units of lipase, 2,500 international units of amylase, and 300 international units of protease, plus 500 to 1,000 milligrams of pancreatin, immediately after the two largest meals of the day to ensure complete digestion.
Note: Long-term supplementation with pancreatin is not advised, as it can cause your pancreas to reduce its own production of this important enzyme. Overuse also has the potential to cause nausea or diarrhea. After two months on pancreatin, discontinue use and monitor your reaction. If you find that your digestive problems recur, discuss pancreatin supplementation with your health-care provider.

Indigestion Home Remedies #3: Glutamine can help soothe irritation in the gastrointestinal tract. Try taking 500 milligrams of L-glutamine two to three times daily for up to one month.

Indigestion Home Remedies #4: Take probiotic supplements of acidophilus and/or bifidobacteria. For indigestion, powdered or liquid formulas are the best choice; these work in the stomach, while capsules open in the intestines. Tablets are not usually as effective, and must be chewed thoroughly.

Indigestion Home Remedies #5: Acidophilus powder can be taken any time for indigestion—simply take 1/4 to 1/2 teaspoon as needed. If you must use capsules, open them and pour the contents onto your tongue rather than swallowing them whole. If you are allergic to milk, select a dairy-free formula.

Indigestion Home Remedies #6: Vitamin E soothes the stomach. Choose the mixedtocopherol or d-alpha tocopherol form, not dl-alpha-tocopherol. Begin by taking 200 international units daily and gradually increase the dosage until you are taking 400 international units once or twice daily.
Note: If you have high blood pressure, limit your intake of supplemental vitamin E to a total of 400 international units daily. If you are taking an anticoagulant (blood thinner), consult your physician before taking supplemental vitamin E.

HERBAL TREATMENT FOR INDIGESTION

Indigestion Home Remedies #7: Aloe vera juice helps to clear and resolve an upset stomach that feels "burning." Make sure to get a food- grade product. Take 1 tablespoon diluted in 6 ounces of water up to three times daily. Use it sparingly; it can be a strong cathartic.

Indigestion Home Remedies #8: Gentian root is a bitter herb that has been used for centuries throughout Europe to enhance digestion, especially of proteins and fats. Take 500 milligrams twice a day, with meals.

Indigestion Home Remedies #9: Ginger is a notable digestive aid. It aids digestion, enhances assimilation, and reduces nausea. Take one or two 500-milligram capsules as needed.

Indigestion Home Remedies #10: Deglycyrrhizinated licorice (DGL) can be amazingly helpful. Chew two 250- to 500-milligram lozenges with a glass of water twenty minutes before each meal.
Note: Ordinary licorice can elevate blood pressure, and should not be taken on a daily basis for more than five days in a row. DGL should not have this effect, however.

Indigestion Home Remedies #11: Peppermint is a time-tested, time-honored herb that is very effective for all forms of indigestion. It enhances digestion, speeds the emptying time of the stomach, and reduces flatulence. Drink peppermint tea with meals.
Note: If you are using peppermint tea and also taking a homeopathic preparation, allow one hour between the two. Otherwise, the strong smell of the mint may interfere with the action of the homeopathic remedy.

An abscess is a local accumulation of pus. It can occur almost anywhere on or in the body, but it most frequently occurs on the skin and on the gums of the mouth. Abscesses can be very tender and painful and are marked by inflammation, swelling, heat, redness, and often fever. Abscesses are caused by an infection, so orthodox medical doctors often treat them with antibiotics. But herbs are an effective and safe alternative, without the side effects of antibiotics.

Abscess Home Remedies #1:
SKIN-ABSCESS—FIGHTING TEA
3o drop echinacea tincture
6o drop.a yerba mania tincture
1 cup warm water
Combine all the ingredients. Take up to five times per day to stimulate the immune system and help eliminate the infection.

Abscess Home Remedies #2:
TOPICAL WASH FOR SKIN AND GUM ABSCESSES
1 to 2 teaspoons barberries
1 tablespoon white oak bark
1 teaspoon echinacea root
1 teaspoon granulated Oregon grape root
2 cups boiling water
Combine the herbs in a glass container. Pour the boiling water over the herbs and soak for 3 to 4 hours; strain. Use three times a day as a wash. If you are using this tea to treat a gum abscess, be sure to swish the liquid around in your mouth for several minutes before spitting it out.

DIETARY GUI IELINES FOR ABSCESS

Abscess Home Remedies #3: Drink at least ten 8-ounce glasses of pure water daily until the abscess heals.

Abscess Home Remedies #4: Eat plenty of steamed leafy green vegetables and sea vegetables to ensure a good supply of vitamins and minerals needed for healing.

Abscess Home Remedies #5: Eat fresh pineapple. Fresh pineapple contains bromelain, which is very effective at reducing inflammation.

Abscess Home Remedies #6: Eliminate from your diet all fried foods and anything containing refined sugar, which slow healing.

NUTRITIONAL SUPPLEMENTS FOR ABSCESS

Abscess Home Remedies #7: Blue-green algae contains many trace minerals that are needed for healing and that are missing in the average diet. Take 300 milligrams two or three times daily.

Abscess Home Remedies #8: Colloidal silver is a liquid mineral supplement that fights infection. Take 10 drops three to four times daily

Abscess Home Remedies #9: If you must take antibiotics, restore the body's "friendly" bacteria by taking a probiotic supplement, such as acidophilus and/or bifidobacteria, as recommended on the product label. If you are allergic to milk, select a dairy-free formula. Colostrum is another effective probiotic that can be taken on a rotating basis with acidophilus and bifidobacteria. Take 300 milligrams three times daily, between meals.

Abscess Home Remedies #10: Vitamin C and bioflavonoids improve the immune response and help to reduce inflammation. Take 1,000 milligrams of vitamin C three to five times daily and 500 milligrams of mixed bioflavonoids three to four times daily.

HERBAL TREATMENT

Abscess Home Remedies #11: Cat's claw enhances the immune response and has antibacterial properties. Take 500 milligrams of standardized extract three times a day until the abscess clears.
Note: Do not use cat's claw if you are pregnant or nursing, or if you are an organ-transplant recipient. Use it with caution if you are taking an anticoagulant (blood thinner).

Abscess Home Remedies #12: Echinacea and goldenseal have antibacterial properties and also boost the body's natural immune response. They are helpful for fighting virtually any type of infection. Take one dose of an echinacea and goldenseal combination formula supplying 250 to 500 milligrams of echinacea and 150 to 300 milligrams of goldenseal three to four times daily for up to one week.

While any excessive or unusual bleeding is certainly a medical emergency, herbs can also be very effective for bleeding from a wide variety of causes.

Traditionally these anti-hemorrhagic herbs are called styptics. Indeed, their unique ability to both prevent and arrest bleeding should make them part of every emergency kit. Botanical medicines can work speedily for bleeding from injuries or wounds. They are also very effective for ruptures of capillaries or small veins in the nose, gums or around hemorrhoids.

Several herbs are particularly effective as a compress, wash or lotion for these types of external bleedings, especially calendula, St. John's wort and witch hazel. These vulnerary herbs also have the advantage of accelerating wound healing, while being antiseptic. Additionally, herbs rich in collagen-building nutrients, bioflavonoids and vitamin C can strengthen blood vessels to prevent excess bruising or bleeding. Other plants are effective for internal bleeding as well, affecting organs that include the stomach, intestines and bronchial tubes. Geranium, lesser periwinkle and lady's mantle are good examples. Excess menstrual bleeding (menorrhagia) or bleeding between periods (metrorrhagia) require attention and specific herbs such as trillium and shepherd's purse. Naturally, any underlying causes of bleeding, such as hormonal imbalance, need to be discovered and dealt with. See also Anemia - Cuts -Menopause

Home remedies for Bleeding

Home remedies for Bleeding #1: Calendula**—Marigold/Calendula officinalis
· Stops bleeding from wounds, or from the scalp, mouth or gums.
· For external use on wounds, scrapes, cuts. Antiseptic and disinfectant, while accelerating tissue healing and prevents secondary infection.

Home remedies for Bleeding #2: Cayenne***—Capsicum frutescens
· Extract or powder applied externally stops bleeding in small wounds.
· Speeds healing by improving circulation and has antiseptic effects.
· Capsules or tea reduce internal bleeding. Useful for nosebleeds.

Home remedies for Bleeding #3: Geranium**—Cranesbill/Geranium maculatum
· An astringent and styptic; decreases clotting time in external wounds.
· Especially for bleeding in the digestive tract, including stomach ulcers, bleeding and diarrhea in irritable bowel syndrome or Crohn's disease.
· May also be used in excess menstrual or vaginal bleeding.

Home remedies for Bleeding #4: Lady's Mantle*—Alchemilla vulgaris
· Promotes blood coagulation and is a strong astringent for internal bleeding, heavy menstrual flow or bloody diarrhea.
· Useful as a rinse after dental surgery or as a douche for vaginitis.

Home remedies for Bleeding #5: Lesser Periwinkle**—Vinca minor
· Astringent/styptic for internal bleeding, bloody diarrhea or heavy menses.
· Reduces bleeding from nose, gums, mouth or after tooth extractions.
· Useful for arteriosclerosis and insufficient blood flow to the brain.

Home remedies for Bleeding #6: Raspberry Leaf*—Rubus idaeus
· Traditional use to prevent or treat bleeding during pregnancy or labor.
· Used to stop bleeding from skin ulcers, wounds, gums or sore throat.
· An effective astringent used to treat conjunctivitis, diarrhea, vaginitis.

Home remedies for Bleeding #7: Shepherd's Purse***—Thlaspi bursa pastoris
· A strong styptic; stops bleeding from external wounds, nosebleeds.
· Internally for bloody diarrhea and dysentery or urinary tract bleeding.
· Used for heavy uterine bleeding during or between menses or due to fibroids, miscarriage, menopause or post-partum bleeding.

Home remedies for Bleeding #8: St. John's Wort***—Hypericum perfoliatum
· Stops bleeding from injuries and open wounds, puncture wounds, abrasions, irritated gums or hemorrhoids (take internally and externally).
· Internally: effective for various kinds of bleeding or bleeding tendency.
· Externally: antiseptic and antiviral, speeds healing of wounds, burns.

Home remedies for Bleeding #9: Trillium***—Birthroot/Trillium erectum or pratense
· Excellent for excess bleeding associated with fibroids, too frequent or prolonged periods, bleeding between periods or uterine prolapse.
· Specific benefit for excess blood loss during menopause.
· Uterine tonic; relieves pain in the back, hip and pelvis.

Home remedies for Bleeding #10: Witch liazel***—Hamamehs virginiana
· Apply to wounds, cuts, nosebleeds, or for injury to veins, eyes.
· Good for chronic effects of trauma, for bruising; relieves pain, soreness.
· Stops bleeding, prevents infection, promotes healing in ragged wounds.

Home remedies for Bleeding #11: Yarrow***—Achillea millefolium
· An astringent healing herb, effective for hemorrhage from wounds, internal injuries, hemorrhoids, after surgery or childbirth, nosebleed.
· Internal use to staunch bleeding from lungs, bladder, bowels, uterus.
· Specifically benefits endometriosis, bleeding from varicose veins.
Note: Other astringents that arrest bleeding include oak, bistort and plantain. For hormone-related bleeding, consider vitex, rnaca and especially clong quai to regulate menses.

Cramping Home Remedies

Cramping can occur in any hollow organ of the body, but here we are primarily dealing with spasms in the digestive tract. Causes are many, including indigestion, infection or inflammation anywhere in the intestinal tract. Infantile colic, due to weak digestion, food allergies and gas formation, is a trial for both mother and baby. In adults, a variety of irritants can cause acute cramps, while chronic gut toxicity causes cramps relating to dysbiosis, irritable bowel and colitis. In all cases, underlying causes need to be addressed while painful spasms are being alleviated.

Antispasmodic herbs can provide a simple and non-toxic approach to calming painful cramps and colic. Such herbs are often nervines as well, providing sedative and calming effects for jangled nerves.

Other needed herbs are also carminatives, helping expel excess gas, and digestive tonics with anti-inflammatory effects. Deeper problems can be improved with herbal detoxification programs for the intestines and liver. In colic, food allergies in the baby, or in a mother who is breastfeeding, need to be identified and eliminated, until the immune system can be re-regulated to eliminate these sensitivities. The same holds true for adults.

Cramping Home Remedies

Home remedies for cramp #1: Anise***—Pimpinella anisum
· An important infant and child remedy for colic and general cramping.
· Antispasmodic and carminative, eases nausea, indigestion, bloating.
· Safe, gentle, tasty; can work via the breast milk. Improves appetite.

Home remedies for cramp #2: Caraway**—Carum carvi
· Similar to fennel and anise, relieves intestinal colic or cramps associated with gas, bloating, digestive upset, nausea and indigestion.
· Gentle enough for children, also good for menstrual cramping.

Home remedies for cramp #3: Catnip***—Nepeta cataria
· Relieves intestinal spasm and gas, diarrhea; mild relaxing effect.
· Relieves upset stomach, indigestion. Safe in children and the elderly.
· Is especially effective for intestinal or gastric upset of a nervous origin.
· Gentle and calming; sedates anxiety, reduces fever, eases headaches.

Home remedies for cramp #4: Chamomile***—Matricaria recutita
· Effective antispasmodic and colic remedy, soothes indigestion; anti- inflammatory and antiseptic. Calms irritability, restlessness, insomnia.
· Antidotes effects on nursing child of coffee or drug use by mother.

Home remedies for cramp #5: Cramp Bark***—Viburnum opulus
· Stronger antispasmodic than black haw; relieves painful cramping in

abdomen, stomach, uterus or bladder. Relieves back pain, neuralgia.
· Effective for menstrual cramps, false labor pains. Helps with leg cramps.

Home remedies for cramp #6: Dill***—Anethum graveolens
· Relieves intestinal spasms, cramps, infantile colic and indigestion.
· Dispels gas and calms and improves the digestion; antibacterial action.
· Increases breast milk, which carries antispasmodic effects to the infant.

Home remedies for cramp #7: Fennel**—Foeniculum vulgare
· Stimulates digestion, relieves colic, flatulence, bloating and distension.
· Like anise and caraway, also used in coughs, as an antispasmodic and expectorant. Increases breast milk; has a reputation as a longevity herb.

Home remedies for cramp #8: Kava Kava**—Piper methysticum
· Muscle relaxant and antispasmodic for internal organs and muscle tension. Sedative pain and cramp reliever, reduces sensitivity to pain.
· Strongly reduces anxiety, relieves sleeplessness, is a mild antiseptic.

Home remedies for cramp #9: Lemon Balm* *—Melissa officinalis
· Eases cramps and spasms, gas and bloating, indigestion and colic pains, gastric acidity. Useful for problems related to stress and anxiety.
· A good children's herb; soothes anxiety, irritability, restlessness.

Home remedies for cramp #10: Licorice**—Glycyrrhiza glabra
· Demulcent and anti-inflammatory, decreases the spasms of gastritis or intestinal distress, relieves stomach ulcers and body's stress response.
· Mild laxative, assists in the body's clearing of poorly digested foods.

Home remedies for cramp #11: Peppermint**—Mentha piperta
· Digestive antispasmodic; relieves colic, spasm, spastic constipation.
· Carminative, dispels gas and distention, with pain-relieving action.
· Stomachic, improves digestion, stimulates secretions and bile output.

Home remedies for cramp #12: Valerian**—Valeriana officinalis
· A sedative and antispasmodic, relaxing intestinal cramps, muscle tension. Relieves spasms and pain related to anxiety and emotional upset.
· For cramps with diarrhea, or after eating. Promotes restful sleep.

Home remedies for cramp #13: Wild Yam***—Dioscorea villosa
· Important antispasmodic for cramps in any hollow organ; intestines, stomach or gall bladder spasm. For colic that is relieved by stretching.
· Helps with gas and flatulence, belching, indigestion, upset from tea.

Home remedies for cramp #14: Yarrow*—Achillea millefolium
· A digestive antispasmodic, anti-inflammatory and pain reliever.
· For cramping pains or stomachache, distension, or gas pain.
· A sedative and tranquilizing herb that promotes tissue healing.

Home Remedies for Rosacea

Rosacea is a skin disease of the small blood vessels of the face. Although it is sometimes called acne rosacea, it is not associated with a previous history of acne. It affects about 5 percent of the population, mostly women who are menopausal and in their forties, especially those who are fair-skinned and of Celtic ancestry. The face, especially the nose and central face, is affected with a symmetrical red rash, with or without prominent fine blood vessels, or telangiectasia. Papules (small, solid bumps), pustules (inflamed, pus-filled bumps) and firm red nodules that look like acne lesions are often scattered over the cheeks and nose as well However, unlike acne, rosacea is not characterized by the formation of blackheads or whiteheads. In some cases, a bulbous red nose, or rhinophyma, may develop slowly if the condition is left untreated.

Many experts believe that the cause of rosacea is infectious a result of infection with skin mites, the yeast Pityrosporum ovale, which is normally present in hair follicles, or with as-yet-unidentified bacteria or fungi. Others think that psychological factors, genetics, and/or connective tissue problems in the skin are the likely cause. Probably a combination of these factors, and possibly others, is responsible.

Many people with rosacea experience blushing or Hushing of the face, especially in hot weather, with sung exposure, and after consuming spicy foods, alcohol, hot drinks or soup, coffee, or tea. These factors, which dilate local facial blood vessels, also worsen the acne-like lesions. Food intolerances, inadequate stomach-acid production, and a deficiency of the 13 vitamins, especially vitamin. Br, arc also thought to worsen the chronic symptoms of rosacea.

Home remedies for Rosacea

Home remedies for rosacea #1:
Beta-carotene, which the body uses to make vitamin A, helps to strengthen capillaries and is healing for the skin. Take 25,000 international units twice daily.

Home remedies for rosacea #2: The B vitamins, especially vitamin B2 (riboflavin), are necessary for healthy skin, hair, and nails. Take a vitamin-B complex containing 100 milligrams of most of the major B vitamins daily.

Home remedies for rosacea #3: Vitamin C raises immunity, promotes healing, and strengthens connective tissue. Bioflavonoids are anti-inflammatory and help to strengthen blood vessels, and work with vitamin C. Take 500 milligrams of vitamin C with bioflavonoids three times a day

Home remedies for rosacea #4: Zinc also helps to heal the skin. Take 25 milligrams twice a day, with meals and with 1 milligram of copper.

Home remedies for rosacea #5: Flaxseed oil supplies essential fatty acids that help to reduce inflamma tion. Take 1,000 milligrams or 1 teaspoon three times a day

Home remedies for rosacea #6: Acidophilus and bifidus help to restore "friendly" bacteria. If you are taking antibiotics, take either of these supplements as directed by the manufacturer.

Home remedies for rosacea #7: Betaine and hydrochloric acid promote healthy digestion. If you suspect your stomach-acid levels are not high enough, take this supplement as directed by the manufacturer.

HERBAL TREATMENT FOR ROSACEA

Home remedies for rosacea #8: Cat's-claw extract helps to reduce food sensitivities by reestablishing a healthy intestinal environment. Take 500 milligrams three times a day. Caution: Do not take this herb if you are pregnant, nursing, or on blood thinners, or if you are an organ transplant recipient.

Home remedies for rosacea #9: Gotu kola extract promotes healing of the skin. Take 100 milligrams three times a day.

Home remedies for rosacea #10: Grapeseed extract is an anti-inflammatory and antioxidant, and helps in collagen formation. Take 50 milligrams three times a day.

Home remedies for rosacea #11: Some people with rosacea report that horse-chestnut cream or-rose-wax cream is helpful. Either of these products can be applied to the affected areas twice a day.

Home remedies for rosacea #12: Jigucao is a Chinese herbal patent medicine that may be very effective. Take 500 milligrams three times a day.

Home Remedies to Stop a Bleeding Nose

There are a great many tiny blood vessels in the delicate lining of the nose. These small capillaries are easily broken. Any number of things can rupture some of these small vessels and cause a nosebleed.

An accident or assault that results in a blow to the nose can cause your nose to bleed. If you put something in your nose, bleeding can result form the trauma. Even just blowing your nose can start a nosebleed. Inflammation from a cold, an allergy, or dry winter air can cause the vessels to swell and rupture. You may even awaken with blood on your sheets or staining your nightclothes. When a nosebleed occurs from one of these causes, it seldom hurts. More uncomfortable causes include local infection, such as sinusitis, or systemic infections such as scarlet fever, malaria, or typhoid fever.

Blood can be swallowed during a nosebleed, especially one that occurs during the night. If enough blood is involved, you may vomit it up or pass a dark, tarry-looking stool after the nosebleed has stopped.

The blood coming from the nose during a nosebleed can be a continuous stream or a small trickle. It may look as if you are losing a lot of blood, but not much blood is actually lost during the typical nosebleed.

Although a bloody nose, especially one that comes on suddenly and without warning, can be unnerving, nosebleeds can usually be managed easily at home.

Like most wounds, ruptured capillaries inside the nose will heal completely in about ten days.

Certain medical conditions can increase the likelihood of nosebleeds, among them high blood pressure, aplastic anemia, hemophilia, leukemia, Hodgkin's disease, rheumatic fever, thrombocytopenia, and severe liver disease. The use of certain drugs, notably anticoagulants(blood thinners) and aspirin, may be involved as well. Other factors that increase the possibility of nosebleeds include the prolonged use of nose drops, exposure to irritating chemicals, vitamin-C deficiency, high altitude, and a dry climate.

Home remedies to stop a bleeding nose

Home remedies to stop a bleeding nose #1: Vitamin C and bioflavonoids help prevent capillary fragility. Take 500 to 1,000 milligrams of each four times daily for two days after a nosebleed. Then take 500 milligrams of each twice a day for at least one month.

Home remedies to stop a bleeding nose #2: Vitamin K helps the blood to clot more efficiently. If you suffer from recurring nosebleeds, take 25 micrograms once or twice daily for one month.

Home remedies to stop a bleeding nose #3: Another way to stop a nosebleed is to wet a bit of cotton or plain sterile gauze with white vinegar and place it in your nose. Leave it in place for at least ten minutes. The acid of the vinegar will gently cauterize the inside of the nose and stop the bleeding.

How to Stop a Nose Bleed

If you develop a nosebleed, do the following:

1. Calmly sit down in an upright position, not back in the chair. This will help to keep blood from going down the back of your throat. Breathe through your mouth.

2. Tilt your head forward (not backward).

3. Place your thumb and forefinger on either side of the bridge of your nose and pinch the soft part of your nose firmly for ten minutes without releasing. Apply pressure firmly enough to slow bleeding, but not so strongly as to cause discomfort. Pressure decreases the blood flow through the affected area, slowing bleeding. You can also place a cold compress on the bridge of your nose. This has not been proven to be effective but seems to help constrict the local blood vessels.

4. After ten minutes, release the nostrils slowly and check to see if the bleeding has stopped. Avoid touching or blowing your nose. If the bleeding has not stopped, apply pressure for another ten-minute period.

5. If your nose is still bleeding steadily after twenty minutes of pressure, call your health-care provider.

Home Remedies for Bed Sores

Known to doctors as decubitus ulcers, bed sores (or pressure sores) are the result of skin being suffocated beneath the weight of the body. These lesions are caused by continuous extended pressure on the skin, usually in an area over a prominent bone or cartilage structure such as the hips or tailbone.

This pressure restricts the flow of blood, and therefore the supply of oxygen and nutrients, to that part of the skin. Ultimately, the smaller blood vessels clot and a sore red patch of skin appears. If not attended to, it can crack open and develop into a painful wound.

The first sign of a developing pressure sore is reddening of the skin. There may be local swelling or hardening of the tissue as well. Eventually, if the pressure is not relieved, the skin breaks down and ulcerates, and infection may take hold. Obviously, people who are confined to bed for long periods are most at risk for this problem. Wheelchair users also have an increased risk of developing pressure sores.

An individual who suffers from impaired wound healing, common in older adults and people with diabetes, can develop bed sores rather quickly.

When it comes to bed sores, prevention is better than treatment. It is also necessary to rule out the possibility that another disorder might be mimicking a bedsore, especially if the sore appears to be spreading at an unusually fast rate. Herpes lesions, bacterially induced ulcers, and even skin cancers can look like bed sores, but require different treatment.

Home remedies for Bed Sores

Bed Sores Remedies #1: Vitamin C is an anti-inflammatory and is vital for the health of the skin and blood vessels. A study reported in the British Medical Journal found that bedridden patients with bedsores had significantly lower levels of vitamin C in their blood than did similar patients who were free of bedsores. Take 500 milligrams of vitamin C and an equal amount of bioflavonoids three times daily.

Bed Sores Remedies #2: Zinc supports the immune system and promotes wound healing. Take 15 milligrams three times daily. Take zinc with food to prevent stomach upset. If you take over 30 milligrams of zinc on a daily basis for more than one or two months, you should also take 1 to 2 milligrams of copper each day to maintain a proper mineral balance.

HERBAL TREATMENT FOR BED SORES

The following suggestions should be used only if the wound is closed. Open wounds should be attended to by a health-care practitioner.

Bed Sores Remedies #3: Aloe vera, applied topically in ointment, gel, or cream form, is effective in healing sores.

Bed Sores Remedies #4: Topical calendula cream is very soothing and healing to wounds. Use it as directed on the product label.

Bed Sores Remedies #5: Goldenseal is a natural antiseptic; vitamin E is healing and soothing to the skin. Make a paste by combining the contents of three 500-milligram capsules of goldenseal (or 1 teaspoon of goldenseal powder) and 800 international units of vitamin E (pierce capsules and squeeze out the oil). If the resulting mixture is too dry, add a few drops of olive oil. Apply this to the affected area three times daily.

Homemade Remedies For Cough

A cough is a natural reaction, designed to expel irritating, toxic material and mucus accumulations in the bronchial tubes. However, as everyone knows, even repeated coughing is sometimes ineffective at ridding the body of these irritants, and itself become fatiguing and debilitating.

For coughs, there are herbs that have a specific affinity to the chest and lung area (pectorals).

Some herbs are true antitussives or cough-suppressants (coltsfoot, horehound, wild cherry bark, licorice) or are just effective antispasmodics. Many are demulcents, soothing irritated bronchial tubes while others are expectorants, helping expel tough, adherent mucus. The powerful antibacterial and antiviral properties of many of these same plants makes them an excellent choice for getting at both symptoms and causes. Many herbal cough formulas are available that combine these various properties and are often superior to a single herb.

The herbs below represent the best of literally hundreds of herbal cough medicines. Note that demulcent herbs are more applicable to dry coughs (licorice, slippery elm, mullein, althea), while astringent plants are more suitable to moist, rattly or congested coughs (anise, eyebright, cowslip, thyme, eucalyptus). See also Asthma Colds & Flu

Home Remedies for Cough #1:
Anise***—Pimpinella anisum
· Helps expel mucus, while being anti-inflammatory, antispasmodic.
· For colds, coughs, bronchitis; also reduces nausea, gas, bloating.
· Safe for infants and children; a popular colic and indigestion remedy.
· Often mixed with other herbs for above effects and sweet licorice taste.

Home Remedies for Cough #2: Coltsfoot**—Tussilago farfara
· Expels mucus, soothes irritated membranes and suppresses coughs.
· Coughs related to upper respiratory infections (colds), acute and chronic bronchitis, asthma, hoarseness, whooping cough and emphysema.
· See Dosage. Should not be used excessively or for prolonged periods.

Home Remedies for Cough #3: Cowslip**—Primula veris
· Strong antispasmodic and expectorant for rattly coughs, chronic bronchitis with thick white mucus. Warming and sedative effects.

Home Remedies for Cough #4: Elecampane***—Inula helenium
· For coughs and bronchitis, including chronic cough; gentle for children.
· Soothing expectorant; helps expel excess mucus, antibacterial effects.
· Relieves bronchial spasm in asthma, emphysema, bronchitis.

Home Remedies for Cough #5: Eucalyptus**—Eucalyptus globulus
· Expectorant, natural decongestant, often used in rubs and liniments.

· Opens bronchial passages, clears mucus during colds, flu, bronchitis.
· Natural antiseptic. Use as an inhalant or lotion; high toxicity internally.

Home Remedies for Cough #6: Grindella**—Gumweed/Grindelia camporum
· For coughs of bronchitis and asthma, whooping cough or viral coughs.
· Clears tough mucus, improves breathing and smothering tendency on falling asleep. Slows rapid heart beat and reduces high blood pressure.

Home Remedies for Cough #7: Horehound***—Marrubiurn vulgare
· Loosens mucus, soothes coughs; aids stuffy nose, sore throat and colds.
· For bronchitis, wheezing, congested chest, with inability to expel mucus.
· Treats asthma or chronic lung conditions with poor expectoration.

Home Remedies for Cough #8: Hyssop* * *—Hyssopus officinalis
· Relieves coughs, bronchitis; loosens and expels mucus accumulations.
· Best in chronic coughs; a tonic, stimulating herb that speeds recovery.
· Asthmatic coughs in adults, children. Promotes sweat in colds and flu.

Home Remedies for Cough #9: Irish Moss*--Chondrus crispus
· A mucilaginous, jelly-like seaweed used in many respiratory conditions.
· A soothing demulcent used for irritating coughs, inflamed membranes.
· An expectorant for phlegm and mucus, encourages a productive cough.

Home Remedies for Cough #10: Licorice**—Glycyrrhiza glabra
· A powerful cough suppressant, soothing expectorant, demulcent and anti-inflammatory. Treats bronchitis, coughs, asthma, sore throats.

Home Remedies for Cough #11: Lomatium**—Lomatium dissectum
· Powerful antiviral, antibacterial herb, kills at least ten bacterial strains.
· Eliminates a broad range of acute and chronic viruses.
· For flus, cold, chronic bronchitis, viral pneumonia. Expels hard mucus.

Home Remedies for Cough #12: Lungwort* —Sticta pulmonaria
· For cough and bronchitis. For dry hacking night cough, preventing sleep.
· Treats lingering coughs after measles, flu, colds, whooping cough.
· Soothes tickling in throat, bronchi, where one cough incites another.

Home Remedies for Cough #13: Maidenhair Fern*—Adiantum cappillus
· Used for coughs, bronchitis, asthma and general respiratory disorders.
· Soothes sore throats, expels mucus, helps chronic sinus congestion.

Home Remedies for Cough #14: Mullein**—Verbascum thapsus
· Traditional cough remedy that soothes dry and inflamed throat and bronchi, clears mucus, allays bronchial spasms, shrinks swollen glands.
· Useful in colds, flu, bronchitis, asthma and even emphysema.

Homemade Remedies For whitening teeth

We all want white sparkling teeth, just li most movie stars, but let face it; who has the money to buy those expensive systems advertised on TV? and worse yet; who can afford visiting the dentis for one of those laser session that con cost hundreds and hundreds on dollars? Home remedies for whitening teeth are a great alternative for fast, safe and inexpensive teeth whitening.

Home Remedies for whitening teeth #1:
Make a paste by mixing
2 teaspoons of hydrogen peroxide
2 teaspoons of baking soda.
Place the mixture in a small bowl. The thickness of the paste should be consistent as the typical thickness of toothpaste. For a beter taste, add a bit of mint or just a scoop of toothpaste can be combined with the home-made paste for whitening teeth.

Now, how is this home-made whitening theeth remedy re used?

Apply with a toothbrush and leave the mixture on your teeth for at a couple of minutes. You should avoid swallowing the paste. If this happens, just drink lots of water. Use only once or twice a week.

Home Remedies for whitening teeth #1: Brush my teeth really with regular tooth paste. Then pour some extra virgin olive oil on a white wash cloth and scrub your teeth for incredible results

Home Remedies for whitening teeth #2: Make a paste of few drops of lemon juice and a pinch of common baking soda. Apply this to your teeth and massage gently as if brushing. This helps to remove the stain from the teeth.

Home Remedies for whitening teeth #3:
Rub your teeth with the inside of orange peels. Orange peels have a mild compound that has been shown to whiten teeth which removes stains from teeth without damaging the enamel.

IMPORTANT: While hydrogen peroxide is safe to gargle and to use as a home remedy to whitening teeth, one should be extra careful not to swallow any of it as it poses a health hazard to the body. For pregnant or lactating women, any accidental swallowing of the whitening gel could be potentially harmful to the unborn fetus.

When using hydrogen peroxide, you may also experience gum irritation. This is perfectly normal and natural however you should avoid using it if you have any sores inside your mouth.

Home Remedies For Spider Veins

As 75 percent of people over the age of sixty-five know, veins that have become swollen, raised, and snakelike are called Spider Veins. If one or more of the one-way valves in superficial veins no longer functions normally, the blood headed back to the heart can pool or even flow backward. This stretches the vein and makes it impossible for other nearby valves to close properly as well. The vein becomes swollen and kinked, and blood stagnates in the vein. The veins turn purple, dark blue, or cranberry in color.

Spider Veins are most common on the thighs, the backs of the calves, the insides of the legs, and the ankles. In addition to being cosmetically displeasing, Spider Veins often feel heavy, burn, itch, or throb, and the feet and ankles can swell.

The legs may feel hot and heavy and become sensitive to pressure. Symptoms generally worsen during the day, especially with prolonged standing.

The severity of the appearance of the Spider Veins does not necessarily correspond to the severity of the associated pain and soreness.

People with only a few visible varicosities can suffer from severe pain from them.

Spider Veins run in families, and affect women more frequently because of premenstrual or menopausal hormones, birth control pills, and pregnancy. In fact, they occur in 40 percent of pregnant women. Other factors that contribute to Spider Veins include advancing age, muscular atrophy in the legs, poor circulation, smoking, prolonged bed rest, overweight, lack of exercise, prolonged standing or sitting, tight clothing, high heels, excessive heavy lifting, and chronic constipation.

In addition to being painful and tiring, Spider Veins can cause other problems. These include blood clots and inflammation in the veins, and bleeding (either under the skin or on the surface) if the distended vein is accidentally cut or bumped.

The presence of many varicosities prevents the delivery of enough nutrients and oxygen to the tissues of the legs and delays removal of wastes from leg tissues. Then the skin around the varicosities may become very thin, discolored, hardened, and prone to ulcers.

Very tiny dilated capillaries, usually on the face, legs, and thighs, are called spider veins. They are typically a red or bluish color and can be short unconnected lines or come together in a "sunburst" pattern or a spiderweblike pattern just under the surface of the skin. They are not an early sign of Spider Veins and are not a dangerous problem.

Spider veins often run in families, and tend to be more common in women, especially with the hormonal changes of puberty and pregnancy.

Injury to a part of the body or wearing tight hosiery may bring out unwanted spider veins in the involved area. Spider veins also occur on the face in those with fair skin, rosacea, and chronic, unprotected sun exposure.

Home remedies for spider veins

Home remedies for spider veins #1: Horse-chestnut seed offers perhaps the best herbal relief for the swelling, pain, itching, fatigue, and tenseness associated with varicose and spider veins. Clinical studies show that horse chestnut improves circulation in the legs, decreases inflammation, and strengthens the capillaries and veins. Combine ten parts distilled witch hazel with one part tincture of horse chestnut and apply this mixture externally to the affected areas as needed to help ease discomfort. Look for an extract of horse chestnut that provides a daily dosage of 50 milligrams of aescin, one of the key compounds that strengthens capillary cells and reduces fluid leakage. You can also take 500 milligrams of oral horse chestnut three times a day. It usually takes about 3 months to see benefits, so be patient.
Caution: Do not exceed the recommended oral dosage of horse chestnut extract, because larger doses can be toxic.

Home remedies for spider veins #2: Bilberry extract stimulates new capillary formation, strengthens capillary walls, and enhances the effect of vitamin C in reducing blood-vessel fragility. Take 20 to 40 milligrams three times a day.

Home remedies for spider veins #3: Butcher's broom extract improves varicosities by constricting and strengthening veins. Take 300 milligrams three times a day.

Home remedies for spider veins #4: Gingko biloba extract enhances tissue oxygenation and circulation. Take 40 milligrams three times a day.

Home remedies for spider veins #5: Grapeseed extract also improves circulation. Take 50 milligrams three times a day.

Home remedies for spider veins #6: Gotu kola extract is helpful for venous insufficiency, water retention in the ankles, foot swelling, and varicose veins. Take 200 milligrams three times a day.

Home remedies for spider veins #7: Hawthorn extract contains vitamin C, bioflavonoids, zinc, and sulfur, all of which are helpful for varicose veins. Take 200 milligrams three times a day

Home remedies for spider veins #8: Distilled witch hazel is soothingly astringent when applied to areas with varicosities by means of a cotton ball dipped in the extract. Several studies in animals have shown that witch hazel helps to strengthen blood vessels as well.

Supplements for Spider Veins

Vitamin C, bioflavonoids, and vitamin E help to improve circulation and reduce pain from varicosities. Bioflavonoids also strengthen venous walls and connective tissue that supports blood vessels, and vitamin E also acts as a blood thinner to improve circulation. Take 1,000 milligrams of vitamin C and 300 milligrams of a bioflavonoid complex three times daily, and 200 international units of vitamin E twice daily. Take an additional 1,000 milligrams of rutin daily.

Essential fatty acids also help to decrease pain from varicose veins. Take 500 to 1,000 milligrams of black currant seed, borage, or evening primrose oil a day to reduce pain.

Take 25,000 international units of beta-carotene daily.

Take a vitamin-B complex plus an additional 60 milligrams of vitamin B6 daily for several months.

Herbs and Skin Care.

From the Egyptian Queen Cleopatra to the Japanese geishas, all used herbs to protect and rejuvenate their skin, and until the end of the 19th century, for women, herbs were the most important part of the process of looking young and healthy. Their cosmetic tools were natural oils extracted carefully from plants that their mothers had used for the same purpose.

By the middle of the 20th century, the use of herbs was regarded as old fashioned, and we were told that the best products to use for the care of our skin were the ones made in a chemical laboratory. Petrochemicals were blossoming and big corporations started to bombard the public with clever advertising, making them believe that their new synthetic and chemical fill creams were the most effective way of skin care. That's how we forgot that plants were used for hundreds of years to treat skin disorders and to keep it beautiful and healthy.

Looking at the labels of some of these products manufactured by chemists makes me wonder who in their right mind would dare to open the container and spread the content on their faces. Some moisturizers and lotions contain Propylene, glycol, isopropyl and myristate as active ingredients, and that's not all, to get rid of the nasty smell of these chemicals. The manufacturer adds fragrances made from petroleum, the same substance that makes your car run.

You may be using a shampoo or cream that contains herbs and the label reads "natural." Here is a tip, never believe the front label, believe what they are obligated by law to show on the label placed on the back of the container. All ingredients must be listed in a descending order, for example, if the front label reads "Primrose Shampoo" and the back label lists primrose near the bottom, then that product contains very little of the essential oil and chances are that chemicals like hexachlorophene, diazolidinyl and polyquarterium-10, nullify the effectiveness of any botanical substance they may contain. In addition, it has been shown that these chemicals produce wrinkles, but don't worry they also sell creams for that too.

Many people are becoming wary of the adverse effects of chemically produced cosmetics, and you are one of them, that's why you are reading this book, you want to find an alternative. The idea of chemicals in your body is getting old and outdated and since they came to the market there has not been a change for the better. To the contrary, cosmetic surgeries are on the rise. If these products are so amazingly perfectly designed to protect and to prevent, why do we need so much cosmetic surgery?

Skin Care the Natural Way.

Our skin and hair can have different needs, that's why you should choose a preparation that matches your skin complexion and hair type. However, remember that your skin is a reflection of your general health, if you smoke, drink alcohol, or if you have hormonal fluctuations, poor diet, and don't exercise, chances are that your skin will show signs of damage that normal skin treatment will not repair.

To maintain a radiant complexion and healthy hair, eat a balance diet, reduce stress, also rest and relax as much as possible, exercise and use the herb preparations we recommend. All this will ensure that a sufficient blood supply is reaching the layers of the skin, which provides nutrients and oxygen needed to repair and generate new healthy skin tissue.

Herbs can provide all you need to care for your skin. In the next section you'll find some examples of the different properties of herbs and the way to use them.

DRY SKIN PREPARATIONS.

TIP: Did you know that yogurt, placed on the face helps bring water from the deeper layers of the skin to the surface, thus moisturizing your skin for the rest of the day?

Cleanser for Dry Skin.

2 ounces aloe vera gel.
1 tsp. Vegetable oil or jojoba oil or Saint John's Wort oil.
1 tsp. Glycerin.
½ tsp. Grapefruit seed extract.
8 drops Sandalwood essential oil.
4 drops rosemary essential oil.
Mix all ingredients and shake well before use. Apply with cotton balls and rinse with warm water.

Toner for Dry Skin.

Toners are used to improve the appearance of the skin, to soothe and to nourish. Men can use toners as aftershaves.

2 ounces aloe vera gel.
2 ounces orange-blossom water.
1 tsp. wine vinegar.
6 drops rose geranium essential oil.
4 drops sandalwood essential oil.
1 drop chamomile essential oil. *
800 UI vitamin E oil. (Puncture a gel capsule with a needle)
Mix all ingredients and shake well before use.
*The director of the Dermatologic Clinic at the University of Bonn, Germany found that chamomile cream gives a smooth, healthy appearance to rough, red skin faster than other creams and it also reduces the appearance of wrinkles.

Cream for Dry Skin.

3/4 ounces beeswax, shaved. (do not use paraffin)
1 cup vegetable oil.
1 cup of distilled water.
800 UI vitamin E (from a liquid gel)
24 drops rose geranium essential oil.
Heat beeswax and oil in a pot until beeswax melts (it should be warm enough to the touch but without discomfort). In a separate pot heat water until is warm to the touch. Remove the center part of your blender's lid and pour the water in. Turn the blender on high speed and slowly but steadily add the oil and wax mixture. The whole concoction should begin to solidify. Keep adding oil until the mixture does not take any more. Turn off the blender and using a spatula, place the cream in a wide mouthed container.

Facial Steam for Dry Skin.

3 cups of water.
1 drop rose geranium essential oil.
1 drop rosemary essential oil.
1 drop fennel essential oil.
1 drop peppermint essential oil.
Boil water, turn off heat and add essential oils. Place a towel over your head and over the pot, close your eyes and let the steam warm your face. After 15 minutes splash your face with cool water.

Facial Scrub for Dry Skin.

2 tbsp. Oatmeal.
1 tbsp. Cornmeal.
1 tsp. chamomile flowers.
1 tsp. lavender flowers.
1 tsp. elder flowers.
6 drops lavender essential oil.
Grind all dry ingredients in an electric coffee grinder, add essential oil and mix thoroughly. To use, place a small amount of the mixture on the palm of your hand and moisten with a few drops of water to create a paste, wet your face and apply scrub gently. Rinse with warm water.

OILY SKIN PREPARATIONS.

TIP: Did you know that strawberries ans strawberry leaves reduce the production of oil? Other herbs that have a similar effect are basil, eucalyptus, cedarwood, sage, lemon, and ylang-ylang.

Cleanser for Oily Skin.

2 ounces witch hazel.
1 tsp. vinegar.
1 tsp. glycerin.
½ tsp. grapefruit seed extract.
6 drops lemon essential oil.
2 drops cypress essential oil.
Mix all ingredients and shake well before use. Apply with cotton balls and rinse with warm water.

Facial Steam for Oily Skin.

3 cups of water.
1 drop of chamomile essential oil.
1 drop of lemongrass essential oil.
1 drop of lavender essential oil.
1 drop of rosemary essential oil.
Boil water, turn off heat and add essential oils. Place a towel over your head and over the pot, close your eyes and let the steam warm your face. After 15 minutes splash your face with cool water.

Toner for Oily Skin.

2 ounces witch hazel.
1 tbsp. aloe vera gel.
5 drops cedarwood essential oil.
3 drops lemon essential oil.
1 drop ylang-ylang essential oil.
Mix ingredients. Shake well before using.

MATURE SKIN TREATMENTS

The question is, why does skin wrinkle? As you grow older, your body produces fewer of the hormones that keep skin healthy and supplies less oil, protein and natural moisturizing factors which attract and hold water in the skin. This process tends to make the skin drier. As time goes by, collagen and elastin (fibers arranged in a mesh-like pattern) eventually lose their strength, leaving the skin without underlying support and causing it to wrinkle and sag.

Any person over 25 years of age has mature skin, lines start to form around age 30, if you smoke or spend too much time in the sun your skin will look older. Since mature skin does not produce as much oil and natural moisturizers, you will need to follow many of the treatments for dry skin. Herbs can be very important contributors to the development of new cells and several herbs like lavender, neroli, rosemary, rose, and fennel, have been nicknamed centuries ago "anti-aging herbs".

Antioxidants are also very important. They prevent the production of free radicals. These free radicals play an important role in all aspects of aging including hardening of the arteries. They are unstable, quickly multiplying molecules, which are increased by cigarette smoking and other pollutants. Many herbs and vitamins have antioxidant properties and are very powerful in stopping free radicals on their tracks. Some antioxidant herbs are gingko, witch hazel, and essential oil of rosemary, marjoram, and lavender.

Age Spot Remover.

1 tsp. grated horseradish root.
½ tsp. lemon juice.
½ tsp. vinegar.
3 drops rosemary essential oil.
Mix ingredients. Keep away from eyes. Apply as needed on affected areas.

Toner for Mature Skin.

2 ounces aloe vera gel.
2 ounces orange blossom water.
1 tsp. vinegar.
6 drops rose geranium essential oil.
4 drops frankincense essential oil.
4 drops carrot seed essential oil.
800 IU vitamin E oil.
Mix ingredients, apply as needed.

Blemish Remover.

1/4 cup of water.
1 tsp. Epson salts.
4 drops lavender essential oil.
Small cloth.
Mix water and salts, once the salts has dissolved, add lavender. Soak a cotton cloth and compress on affected area. When cloth cools soak it again and repeat several times.

TOOTH DECAY

Tooth decay occurs when a bacteria called streptococcus mutans combined with food debris creates a sticky substance called plaque. This begins to eat away the sugar accumulated between the teeth producing an acid. In turn this acid erodes the teeth destroying calcium and phosphate. The enamel is the first part of the tooth to suffer damage, then the dentin. If left unchecked the damage can go further into the pulp of the tooth where the nerve is causing toothache and infection.

People who consume, too many carbohydrates are at risk of developing tooth decay. Although tooth decay does not show any symptoms until the condition is in the late stages, some sensitivity may develop to cold or hot substances.

Tooth decay requires professional treatment but herbs can help prevent the damage and stop the pain after and before the visit to the dentist.

We recommend

* Take Calcium 1500 mg a day to protect and build strong teeth.

* Vitamin K prevents tooth decay.

* Vitamin D3 helps gum healing and calcium absorption.

TIP: An easy and old way to make a toothbrush is by peeling the bark off one end of a licorice root and flaying the fibres, Marshmallow and cloves can be used as well. This is a good way of brushing your teeth while camping or if you lose your toothbrush since the root has many properties you won't even need toothpaste.

* If you are suffering from toothache, chew some cloves. They are rich in the analgesic oil eugenol. You can soak a piece of cotton in clove oil and place it on the tooth.

* Peppermint is another analgesic but not so strong as cloves.

* Alcohol free Goldenseal extract can be used to kill bacteria and reduce inflammation. Place a few drops on a piece of cotton and keep on the affected tooth overnight.

Inflammation Control Rinse.

2 tsp. dried sage leaves.
1 tsp. kava kava.
1 tsp. St. John's Wort.
2 tsp. White willow bark.
2 cups of boiling water.
Steep for 30 minutes and strain. Use to rinse your mouth several times a day. It reduces inflamation and relieves pain.

* Tooth decay can be caused by acidic saliva. If this is your case, eat lots of raw fruits and vegetables because the minerals found in these foods help keep acidic saliva under control.

* Thyme is a natural antiseptic that reduces the level of bacteria in the mouth.

TIP: Did you know that researchers are looking into adding cranberry extract to toothpastes and mouthwash? Tests results have shown that a compound present in cranberries reduces plaque formation.

Make You Own Mouthwash.

Mix the following ingredients:
20 drops Goldenseal tincture.
20 drops Thyme tincture.
20 drops Myrrh or Echinacea tincture.
10 drops Bloodroot tincture.
4 cups of vodka.

5 cups of water.
5 cups of fresh cranberry juice or 30 drops of cranberry extract.

Shake well before use. If you have used a commercial mouthwash before you know that it cannot be swallowed and it cannot be used by children less than 12 years of age. However, this mouthwash is completely safe for children and although it should not be swallowed, it's not poisoning and it's a lot cheaper than Scope or Listerine.

Your major investment is buying the tinctures but once you have them you can make gallons of mouthwash before you have to buy again. You'll love the taste and the peace of mind knowing that your children are safe.

TIP: Did you know that chewable vitamin C supplements can erode tooth enamel?

Gingivitis

Gingivitis is a common infection of the surface tissue of the gums, caused by a lack of oral hygiene and inappropriate diet. The herbal antimicrobials Echinacea, Eucalyptus, and Myrrh can be used and they are very powerful in the form of tinctures. Depending on the severity of the infection, you can either wash the gums daily with Myrrh tincture or mix equal amounts of Echinacea and myrrh tincture if a stronger remedy is needed. Eucalyptus oil can be used alternately. Use the mouthwash recipe twice a day to kill germs and bacteria.

* Tea tree oil Destroys bacteria, and fungi, responsible for mouth ulcers, gingivitis, canker sores and thrush. Very effective against drug-resistant bacteria. Use a few drops in warm water for an antiseptic gargle.

Pyorrhea

Pyorrhea is a chronic degenerative disease of the gums that must be treated systematically. The treatment consists in using the recommendations for gingivitis with the addition of a high dosage of vitamin C and the following preparation.

Pyorrhea and Abscess Treatment.
Mix the following ingredients:
2 cups Echinacea tea.
1 cup Blue Tag tea.
1 cup Cleavers tea.
1 cup Poke root tea.
Drink 3 times a day for a few weeks or until the condition clears.

Abscess

An abscess is a very painful infection of the mouth. To treat it combine the recommendations for gingivitis and pyorrhea. The preparation shown above will prevent the spreading of the infection to other parts of the mouth.

* Grapefruit Seed Extract is a bacteria killer perfect for mouth infections, ulcers and abscess.

TIP: Did you know that the herb Bloodroot prevents the buildup and removes plaque from teeth, thus preventing tooth decay? Bloodroot is the main ingredient for some over the counter anti plaque mouthwashes.

Mouth Ulcers

Mouth ulcers are very often indicators of one´s general condition and are best treated by improving general health. They commonly occur after the used of antibiotics or during recovery from influenza.

In both cases the body has been exposed to physiological stress resulting in a depressed immune system. This in turn affects the infection fighting capabilities of the mouth resulting in mouth ulcers.

To treat mouth ulcers make a tea using red sage fresh leaves. This is simple and effective. The fresh leaves can also be chewed. Myrrh should be used to kill bacteria and vitamin C and B should be taken as well.

* Grapefruit Seed Extract is a bacteria killer perfect for mouth infection, ulcers and abscess.

* Tea tree oil Destroys bacteria and fungi responsible for mouth ulcers, gingivitis, canker sores and thrush. Very effective against drug-resistant bacteria. Use a few drops in warm water for an antiseptic gargle.

Discovering the Cleaning Power of Herbs

We all know that the chemicals used to clean the house are very dangerous especially when small children are around so you should consider removing harsh chemicals not only from your body but from your home as well. This is very important and I hope everybody would understand the long term effects of pouring dangerous chemicals all over our house, from our counter tops, where we prepare our food, to our toilets and floors.

We should remember that many cleaners and repellents have been removed from the market after it was discovered that certain chemicals in them were causing birth defects, or serious skin disorders, and the truth is that nobody knows for sure when the chemicals that are being used today will be pulled out of the market for similar reasons.

I would like to share with you my personal experience with dangerous chemicals. I was 11 months old when I crawled to the kitchen and opened the cupboard where the bleach was stored. I managed to take the lid off and spill the contents all over my body. My mother who had stepped out of the room for a few seconds, was alerted by my screams and choking sounds. I guess I was very fortunate that the bleach bottle was full and too heavy for me to pick up and drink from it.

Household cleaner ingestion and pesticides related problems cause 18,000 emergency room trips each year. That is why this is not a subject for environmental extremists or chemical sensitive people, the risk and potential danger are so great that consumers are informing themselves and a change is starting to take place. The power of herbs is being rediscovered as the truth about these poisons is uncovered little by little.

Worrying about household chemicals is a relatively new preoccupation. Since World War II, there has been a petrochemical boom. Companies realized these synthetic chemicals could be produced cheaply and in large quantities as active ingredients in household cleaners and personal hygiene products to kill germs and other microorganisms.
All of this sounds very good and useful until you realize that petrochemicals don't discriminate between harmful bacteria and good bacteria or the organisms in our bodies that help us fight infection,

germs, and viruses. The petrochemicals, which turn out to give us a false sense of security and cleanliness, disrupt our body's natural order of balance.

Our grandparents and parents can probably debate us saying that they have used them for years and nothing bad has happened to them. This may be true but they have not been exposed to these chemicals from an early age when the immune system is not at its fullest. This could be one of the reasons why we have so many children with a wide array of allergies and disorders. No one in history has faced the toxic experience confronting our children today.

The National Academy of Science estimates that 15 % of Americans have a chemical sensitivity that affects their quality of life. Experts only expect this number to rise unless we do something to remove these chemicals from our lives.

Before World War II there were no chemicals being used in our homes. Today household cleaners contain about 4,000 toxic chemicals, which can cause long term nerve damage or death if ingested, not to mention the wide array of respiratory and skin disorders caused by everyday exposure to these poisons. Residues from more than 400 toxic chemicals, including a good number from household products, have been found in human blood and fat tissue. The Consumer Product Commission has determined that more than 150 chemicals in ordinary household cleaners have the potential to cause cancer, nerve damage, birth defects, and fertility problems.

The EPA (Environmental Protection Agency) considers indoor air pollution one of the principal threats. EPA says that pollution inside a home can be 3 to 5 times higher than outdoor pollution. Air neutralizers, room deodorizers "plug-ins" all spray harmful synthetic chemicals into the air. In this part of the book we'll show you how to turn your regular "plug-ins" into herbal deodorizers using essential oils. We will go through your house mentioning the products that you may be using now and suggesting the herbal combination that replaces the synthetic chemicals.

We recommend

Oven Cleaner.

½ cup baking soda.
½ cup liquid Castile soap.
7 drops lemon essential oil.
7 drops eucalyptus essential oil.

5 drops lavender essential oil.
1 cup of hot water.
Preheat oven to 225 degrees F, then turn off and leave door open. Combine all the ingredients and pour into a spray bottle. Shake well and spray on oven walls and door, wait for 20 minutes, wipe off, and repeat if necessary.

Kitchen Sink Scrub.

½ cup baking soda.
1/8 cup white vinegar.
5 drops lemon essential oil.
5 drops orange essential oil.
Mix all the ingredients and scrub metal sink using a green scrub pad.

Bath Tub and Shower Scrub.

½ cup baking soda.
10 drops tea tree oil essential oil.
10 drops lavender essential oil.
Mix all ingredients and use to scrub the tub and tiles with a green scrub pad. This mixture will prevent mold and mildew buildup. If the areas are covered by hard-to-get-off mildew, use tea tree oil and water in a spray bottle. Spray over the area every day for a week, then twice a week.

Vacuum Cleaner Deodorizer.

Moisten 3 cotton balls in lavender essential oil and place them in a vacuum cleaner bag to scent the carpets and the air.

Dishwashing Detergent.

Buy a bottle of castile soap.
Add 10 drops of lemon essential oil.
10 drops lavender essential oil.
10 drops orange essential oil.
Shake well before using.

Natural disinfectant.

5 drops lavender essential oil.
5 drops lemon essential oil.
5 drops orange essential oil.
5 drops eucalyptus essential oil.
5 drops tea tree essential oil.
Add oils to a small spray bottle with water. Use it to wipe and disinfect counter tops, tables, stoves.

Closet deodorizer and moths repellent.

Moist a few cotton balls with cedarwood essential oil, eucalyptus essential oil, and pine essential oil. Place the cotton balls in drawers and shelves. This keeps the bugs out and your closet smells like cedar.

Insect repellent.

10 drops eucalyptus essential oil.
5 drops cedarwood essential oil.
5 drops sandalwood oil.
5 drops peppermint essential oil.
2 ounces of Vodka.
5 drops of geranium oil.
Mix all ingredients in a dark glass bottle and use as needed. However, keep away from mouth and eyes because essential oils are powerful and vodka has alcohol in it which can be very annoying if sprayed in someone's mouth or eyes.

Glass Cleaner.

Mix the following:
10 drops of grapefruit essential oil.
10 drops of lemon essential oil.
2 cups of lavender or rubbing alcohol.
1 cup of white vinegar.
How to use: Put all ingredients in a spray bottle and use with paper towel or scrunched up newspaper. It will create a delightful scent in your house when the sun shine warms up your windows.

Floor Cleaner and Polisher.

In bucket full with hot water place:
20 drops of eucalyptus essential oil.
20 drops lemon essential oil.
2 cups of white vinegar.
1/4 cup of castile soap.
This mixture is great for linoleum, tile and wood floors.

Plug Ins Herbal refills.

If you use the plug ins, that come with a small bottle that inserts, on the bottom of the unit, refill the bottle with your favorite essential oil (mine is lavender or cedarwood) and plug it back into the unit. This will keep your home smelling great and you will save money those refills are quite expensive, also you will get peace of mind knowing that your herbal refill does not spray hash chemicals on the air.

1.- Un plug unit from the electrical outlet.

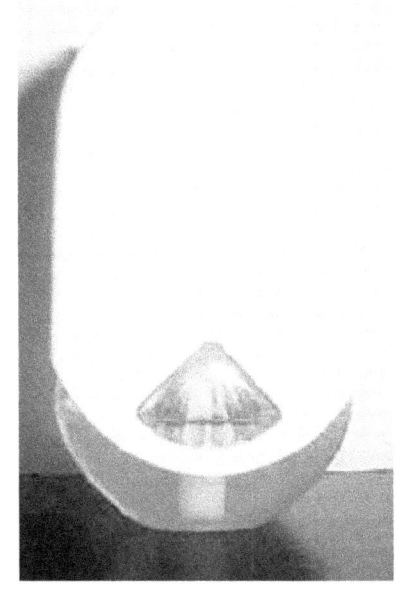

2.-Remove oil container

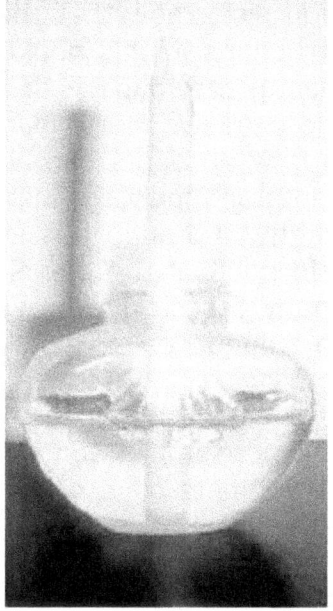

3.- Remove top part and fill with essential oils, replace top part, and insert into the unit.

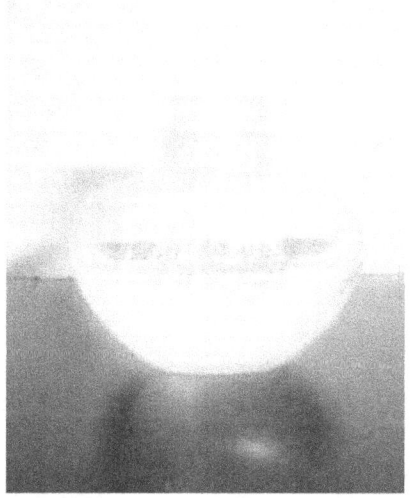

By now you already know that I back what I recommend with research and statistics. You also know that the remedies you are making following the instructions in this book and on www.homemademedicine.com are made with herbs, minerals, and nutrients and that they do work wonders. Many people ask me what I mean by "Nutrients" and how nutrients can heal an illness. Most people believe that nutrients or foods are just to sustain life and to some extend keep us healthy. Although this is true, there are some very powerful properties in most of the plants, spices, and other foods we eat, which in many cases have proven to reduce tumors, unclog arteries, speed up wound healing and much more.

Did you know that heart disease and cancer are the number one killers in the world? Everywhere but in some parts of Italy. Why? Because they include in their diets olive oil and garlic and lots of it.

Not long ago a member of my website wrote to me concerned about her husband's high cholesterol, she was looking for a natural alternative to lower it I recommended that she start including garlic, and almonds into his diet. She was shocked and replied "but I have known for years that almonds increase cholesterol levels"; she was not aware of the latest research done and the newly found compound in almonds that actually lowers cholesterol. So she was not utilizing a very important tool in the fight against high cholesterol.

Misinformation is a very big problem we have faced in the field of natural medicine even doctors and scientist used to dismiss the power of garlic as an "old wives' tales". However, after all the recent research scientist are now taking garlic very seriously and people are starting to use it more and more. In the United States alone more then 5 million people take garlic daily. And in Europe, more specifically in Germany, the Health Ministry has determined that garlic "IS A MEDICINE" that prevents age related deterioration of the circulation.

Information is so powerful and lack of information can be deadly when it comes to your health. If you are not a member of our web site you are missing a big piece of information that can make your life better and the amount of money you will save is also big.

www.homemademedicine.com

A

B

C

D

E

F

G

H

I

L

M

N

O

P

R

S